The XXL Keto Diet Book For Beginners

Quick, Super-Amazing and Delicious Keto Recipes for Everyday Enjoyment I incl. Sides, Snacks, Desserts & More I BONUS: Meal Plan

MATTHEW K. CHARLES

Table of Contents

EXCLUSIVE BONUS

40 Weight Loss Recipes

&

14 Days Meal Plan

Scan the QR-Code and receive
the FREE download:

The Keto Diet: A Beginner's Guide

What Is the Keto Diet?

The ketogenic diet is a low-carb alimentary regimen, which promotes the use of high-fat food. Several studies highlight that this diet can be beneficial for losing weight and improving our overall health.

Following the keto diet means drastically reducing the amount of carbohydrates. These should instead be replaced with fat and protein. This alimentary regimen puts the body into a metabolic state known as ketosis. This means that our body will become more efficient at burning fat and calories, which translates into weight loss.

Different Types of Keto Diet

As a general rule, following the keto diet means reducing the intake of carbs. Nevertheless, there are several versions of this diet, to suit the needs of each body. This includes:

- **Standard Ketogenic Diet.** This is the alimentary regimen that most people follow. The ideal daily intake should contain 75% fat and 20% protein, leaving only 5% or less for carbs.
- **Targeted Ketogenic Diet.** If you are an athlete or you work out often, you may want to introduce carbs before going to the gym.
- **Cyclical Ketogenic Diet.** Some people prefer having 2 days out of 7 when they eat food rich in carbs.
- **High-Protein Ketogenic Diet.** This is a diet particularly rich in protein (about 35% of your daily intake).

What is Ketosis and How Does It Work?

The main aim of the keto diet is to reach the status of ketosis.

This is a process that happens when your body does not have enough carbs to burn to produce energy. This forces our bodies to burn fat. You can start ketosis in just 3 or 4 days if you start eating fewer than 50 grams of carbs per day and fasting.

Research has shown that ketosis has several benefits, which includes weight loss. For example, it can help lower the risk of heart disease, as well as reducing the symptoms of metabolic syndrome and insulin resistance.

How Much Fibre Do I Need?

Doctors recommend 25/31 grams of fibre per day. On the other hand, several studies have shown that eating more fibres can reduce the risk of heart disease and cancer.

To make sure your diet is healthy and adequate for your body, you can start with no more than 20 grams of fibre per day. You can then increase your daily intake if you need to. Don't forget to get your fibre from whole foods.

What Does "Intermittent Fasting" Means?

One of the characteristics of the keto diet is intermittent fasting. This involves periods of fasting and eating. Usually, you should wait up to 6-8 hours between two of your main meals.

Studies have shown that intermittent fasting can provide significant benefits to our health. This includes weight loss and other things.

Remember that the keto diet aims to provide your body with all the macros it needs to sustain intermittent fasting and keep burning calories.

How Does Fasting Work?

When you eat, you are ingesting energy which your body uses immediately. However, part of this energy is stored. This is when your body uses the key hormone known as insulin. In other words, your insulin level rises when you eat.

The energy deriving from carbs is stored in the liver and muscles. The storage here is very limited. This is when the energy turns into excess fat.

This whole process goes in reverse when we are not eating. When you fast, your insulin level falls, and your body starts burning all the stored energy.

The Importance of Tracking Your Macros

People who are on a diet are needed to track their calories. Similarly, if you wish to follow a ketogenic lifestyle, you must track your macros. This is the best way to review your daily intake of carbs so that you can get into ketosis easier and quicker.

To track your macros, you can use a calorie tracking app and your scale. There are many tracking apps available for free on your smartphone or tablet, which will allow you to update your food diary after every meal.

By tracking your macros, you will also feel more motivated, as you will soon understand how easy it is to reduce your intake of carbs and enjoy a healthier lifestyle.

Is Sodium Bad for My Diet?

Many people believe that sodium is bad for our health. This is usually true because a diet rich in carbs means that our levels of insulin are higher. This makes our kidneys retain more sodium.

On the other hand, if you adopt a low-carb lifestyle, your insulin levels will be much lower, meaning that your body will need more salt. Experts suggest adding an extra 3 or 5 grams of sodium in your diet when you are in ketosis.

By introducing the right amount of sodium in your daily diet, you can avoid electrolyte imbalances. You can just sprinkle pink salt or Himalayan salt on your meal or even add it to your water throughout the day. Many ingredients are rich in sodium and low in carbs. This includes:
- Cucumber
- Celery
- Macadamia nuts
- Organic bone broth

Is Exercising Important?

Maintaining a regular exercise schedule is always important for our physical and mental wellbeing. While on the ketogenic diet, exercise can boost your ketone levels and help you burn calories quicker.

When exercising, you help your body deplete its glycogen stores. When your body runs out of those, it will start seeking other forms of energy, and thus switch into ketosis.

To make sure that you are exercising properly, you should find the perfect balance between low-intensity state exercises (such as walking or jogging), and a higher intensity schedule.

Nevertheless, if your body is struggling to get used to your new alimentary regimen, or if you are experiencing the symptoms of the keto flu, you should allow yourself to spend some time away from the gym. You will be ready to go back as soon as your body will start entering ketosis.

While trying to lose some weight and eating healthy food, you should also avoid energy drinks. Even if those often have zero calories, they may still not fit your ketogenic diet plan. Don't forget that they usually contain a high amount of sugar! They will not only jeopardise your diet but also increase your cravings for sweet foods and drinks. You can make your own fruit-infused water at home and, if you want, you can add some sugar substitutes to make them taste sweeter and better.

All the Benefits of a Low-Carb Diet

Many people switch to a low-carb diet to try to lose some weight. Nevertheless, the ketogenic alimentary regimen has many benefits for our body and health. This includes:

- **Losing weight**. Studies have shown that low-carb diets are tendentially more effective than others. Besides, they can even make your body burn more calories than the usual.
- **Reducing symptoms of IBS**. If you suffer from irritable bowel syndrome, the keto diet can help you reduce cramps, pain and even improve your digestion.
- **Better skin** and **less acne**.
- **Lower blood pressure**. Besides, this diet can help reduce your blood sugar, and **potentially reverse type 2 diabetes**.
- A better relationship with food. If you have always suffered from sugar cravings, you know how hard it could be to stay away from sweet food. By following the keto diet, you will still be able to enjoy your favourite treats without feeling guilty.

Potential Side Effects on a Keto Diet

When you decide to stop eating certain foods, your body will need some time to adjust to the new regimen. This is the reason why some people may experience a few side effects in their first month of the keto diet. This may last for a few days or up to two weeks, and side effects may be mild or more stressful depending on how your body is transitioning to your new alimentary choices.

The most common side effect is known as induction flu or keto flu. As soon as you start your low-carb diet, you may experience some of the symptoms of the flu, such as nausea, fatigue, headache, and irritability.

The best way to minimize these symptoms is to drink more fluid. It may also be a good idea to increase your salt intake by drinking a cup of broth one or two times a day.

The keto flu is usually gone after one or two weeks. After this time, you will feel better and you will start enjoying all the benefits of the keto diet!

The Ultimate Keto Shopping List

Meat, Fish and Eggs

Meat, eggs and fish are natural sources of protein, therefore the followings must be regularly consumed if you wish to lose weight with the keto diet.

- Beef
- Pork
- Lamb
- Poultry
- All kinds of fish (preferably fatty ones like salmon)
- Eggs

Vegetables

- Cabbage
- Zucchini
- Asparagus
- Olives
- Mushrooms
- Spinach
- Eggplant
- Cucumber
- Tomatoes
- Peppers
- Lettuce

Dairy Products

You should prefer full-fat options, such as butter, cream and cheeses. Try using butter or cream for cooking, as this will add more natural fat to your meal.

Don't forget to be careful with regular milk, as it usually contains a lot of natural sugar. Preferably, choose coconut, almond or soy milk.

Nuts and Berries
- Brazil nuts
- Almonds
- Macadamia
- Berries (must be eaten in moderation)

Drinks
- Water (still or sparkling)
- Unsweetened coffee or tea
- Wine (in moderation)

Food to Avoid

Starchy Food
- Pasta
- Rice
- Bread
- Potatoes
- French fries
- Porridge
- Muesli

Sugary Food

- Candies
- Juice
- Sports drinks
- Soft drinks
- Cakes
- Pastries
- Chocolate
- Artificial sweetencrs
- Breakfast cereals

Fruit

All fruit except berries.

Starting Your Keto Adventure!

Many people can see the benefits and healthy effects of their new diet after just one month. Nevertheless, your first 4 weeks of the keto diet can be very challenging, as your body will need time to adapt to this new lifestyle.

Don't worry! We have plenty of suggestions to help you go through your first 4 weeks of the keto diet!

Tips to Start Your Keto Diet Like A Pro

- Set a start date for your diet and stick to it.
- Reorganize your pantry and refrigerator before starting your diet and get rid of non-suitable food. By doing this, you won't have any food rich in carbs left at home.
- Make a weekly meal plan, which will also make it easier to buy your food and save some money.
- Get used to reading product labels carefully and always check the ingredients list to spot any hidden carbs.
- Prepare meals ahead of time.
- Drink plenty of fluids, especially if you are in the "keto flu" early stages. Staying hydrated is very important!
- Don't be afraid of temporarily reducing physical activity during the first two weeks of your diet.
- Discuss any doubts or concerns with a doctor before starting your diet or at any time.

How to Start Keto: Week 1

For the first week of keto, it is recommended to allow your body to get used to running without the usual influx of carbs.

The best way to kickstart your diet is to forget about calories and to not constantly check where you are in ketosis.

The first week is all about listening to your body and your mind, and avoiding sugars and carbs. To make it easier, you should:

- **Eat lots of non-starchy veggies**. This includes cauliflowers, broccoli, and green leafy vegetables.
- **Cut out high glycaemic foods**. You should avoid bread, pasta and rice. There are plenty of great substitutions which will make you feel satisfied.
- **Do not exaggerate with proteins**. They are important, but they should be only 15 to 30% of your total intake.

Be prepared for the Symptoms of the "Keto Flu"

During the first few days of your keto diet, you will probably suffer from the "keto flu". This means that you may be experiencing some symptoms that may appear a couple of days after starting a low-carb diet. They may last for up to 1 or 2 weeks.

This includes headache, fatigue, irritability, nausea and constipation. These symptoms are common and should disappear after a few days. You should not become exasperated and frustrated and lose hope. Make sure you drink plenty of water, and you will soon feel better.

Keto Week 2: How to Stay on Your Diet

In week 2 of your keto diet, you should finally get more used to your new alimentary regimen. This means that you should definitely not be eating any pasta, bread, legumes, and grains. Most importantly, the effects of keto flu should now be over.

To ensure that your body keeps adapting to your new diet, you should:
- **Eat fruit once a day**. Always prefer low glycaemic fruits like berries, even though they must be eaten in moderation. Avoid high glycaemic choices, like bananas and watermelons.
- **Go at least 4 hours between meals**. Try to avoid snacks between your main deals, as fasting is essential to achieve ketosis, especially at this stage.
- **Drink plenty of liquid every day**. During this week, hydration is essential, especially to fill your stomach in between meals and avoid eating when you should be fasting.

Keto Diet Week 3: Almost There!

You have finally made it through the first two weeks of your keto diet. You should now feel good and your body should be burning fat rather than carbs.

At this point, you can start testing your ketones to see if you are in ketosis yet. If you are not, you should keep decreasing your carbs. To improve your keto diet, you will need to:
- **Avoid fruit of any type**. Eventually, you will be able to eat a few, small portions of berries, but for now, it is best to cut out all fruit until your body achieves ketosis.
- **Increase fasting**. In week 3, you should try fasting at least 12 hours between your main meals. Of course, you cannot eat any snacks in between. Don't forget that eating causes insulin release. Nevertheless, you can still have plenty of water.

- **Drink more!** Water is your ally in your battle for a healthier body and lifestyle. However, if you get sick of water, you can switch to different options, such as coffee or tea.
- **Start checking your food intake.** You should now be a pro when it comes to keto recipes, and it is thus time to track your macros and write down your food intake. You can use either a diary or more advanced options, such as an app on your smartphone. You don't need to track calories.

Keto Diet Week 4: Congratulations!

Now you are familiar with what you can and can't eat on a keto diet. Most importantly, you should now be able to listen to all your body's signals, and finally, feel better. At this point, your body has probably started burning fat instead of carbs, and you may have already lost some weight.

This means that you shouldn't stop it now, nor that you have already achieved everything you were aiming for. In fact, this is where your diet becomes even more serious!

Tips and Trick to Stick to a Keto Diet

You do not need particular cooking skills to make a low-carb diet and eat healthy food. On the other hand, you may always need a few tips and tricks to stick to your diet and feel better.

Prepare for the Keto Flu

The keto flu is maybe the only negative side of the keto diet. Luckily enough, it only lasts for one week or two.

Although you will not necessarily suffer from it, you must be prepared to experience the keto flu. You may feel dizzy, suffer from nausea or insomnia, and even feel frustrated and unmotivated. Don't worry and try to stick to your new dietary regimen! At the end of this "flu", you will feel better and you will notice that your body is changing. You will start losing weight, and you may experience some of the many benefits of a low-carb diet.

Don't forget to drink plenty of water and consume foods rich in minerals. Mineral supplements may also be helpful, although you should usually try to avoid them.

Breakfast is the most important meal of the day...

.... And it is also the best time to eat low carb. The keto diet is the perfect excuse to enjoy scrambled eggs, bacon and other savoury food without feeling guilty. Nevertheless, there is still a variety of sweets you can prepare and eat for breakfast, such as pancakes and cookies.

If you are not hungry, you don't need to force yourself to eat anything for breakfast. You can just have a cup of tea or coffee without sugar.

Forget Pasta and Rice

Pasta, rice, potatoes and other starchy ingredients are not part of the keto diet. Nevertheless, you will soon realise that you don't need them. There are plenty of great low-carb alternatives, such as cauliflower mash or cauliflower rice, or even fried cabbage.

Once you try them, you will like them better than any other high-carbs alternative.

Remove Temptations

Especially during your first days on a keto diet, it may be difficult to avoid some of your favourite food. Soon, you will learn how to replicate them with healthier, and low-carb alternatives. Meanwhile, you can make your life easier by getting rid of any temptation.

If you live with people who wish to continue eating these foods, you can just store them in a different cupboard or fridge shelf.

Ease into It

No matter how motivated you are: jumping into a new lifestyle can be difficult and your body will need time to adjust to it.

For this reason, you should try to cut out starchy and sugary food gradually. Start by eliminating all sugars first, then you will be ready to say goodbye to complex carbs. When you feel ready, you can cut out starchy veggies and fruit.

It is essential to listen to your body's signals and be patient. If you are not hungry, you shouldn't necessarily eat. Similarly, if you don't feel full after finishing your meal, try drinking some water or brushing your teeth.

Stay Hydrated

Drinking water is always important, but it is even more essential if you are in ketosis. Don't forget that, by avoiding carbs, you will need to find another way to introduce water in your body. Ideally, you should drink up to 2-3 litres of water per day.

Plan Your Meals

It may take a couple of weeks to get used to a new alimentary regimen. You can start making your life easier by planning your meals. This means that you would not spend hours trying to find something to eat, and you will have all the time to enjoy some delicious food.

Usually, planning for a week ahead is a good idea, especially if you have a busy lifestyle. This will also help you buy only the groceries you need, and avoid wasting your time and money. On the other hand, if you like cooking and expressing your creativity in the kitchen, you can just look at the day ahead in the morning.

Find New Friends

The best way to stay motivated is to find other keto dieters. You and your new friends will be able to share your doubts, struggles and concerns, and even your accomplishments. You may even share new recipes.

There are many ways to find new fellow keto dieters, but joining an online group is usually the easiest. There are several communities with hundreds, if not thousands, of members who are always happy to welcome new users and support them on their weight loss journey.

Stick to Your Plan

Unfortunately, you may happen to realise that the keto diet is not right for you. This may be because of some medical condition, or your overall lifestyle. On the other hand, there are several types of ketogenic diets, which you can choose based on your needs.

After the first week of keto, you may experience significant water and weight loss. Nevertheless, your weight loss journey will follow an unpredictable pattern, since you will not be counting calories. There may be weeks where you don't lose anything and other times when your body will change significantly.

If you believe that your results have been stalling for too long, you can make some adjustments to your diet. However, you should never drastically change your lifestyle. For example, if you want to reduce your carbs even more, or even try a different alimentary regimen, you should ease into it. Your body needs time to adjust to any big change. Otherwise, you will feel poorly and you may even lose all the progress you made with your low-carb lifestyle.

EXCLUSIVE BONUS

40 Weight Loss Recipes

&

14 Days Meal Plan

Scan the QR-Code and receive
the FREE download:

Keto Quick & Easy Recipes

Keto Frittata with Spinach

Difficulty: Easy ¦ Calories 661 ¦ Servings 4
Total Carb: 4 g ¦ Total Fat: 59 g ¦ Protein: 27 g

INGREDIENTS

- 8 eggs
- 150 g (5 oz.) shredded cheese
- 225 g (8 oz.) fresh spinach
- 150 g (5 oz.) diced bacon
- 225 ml (1 cup) heavy whipping cream
- Butter
- Salt and pepper

PREPARATION

1. Preheat the oven to 175 C (300 F).
2. Fry the bacon in butter, then add the spinach and stir well.
3. Whisk the cream and eggs together.
4. Pour the egg mixture into a baking dish, and add the bacon, spinach and cheese on top.
5. Bake for ½ hour.

Keto Tomato Baked Eggs

Difficulty: Easy ¦ Calories 204 ¦ Servings 4
Total Carb: 7 g ¦ Total Fat: 16 g ¦ Protein: 9 g

INGREDIENTS

- 900 g (31 oz.) ripe vine tomatoes
- 4 large eggs
- 3 garlic cloves
- 2 tbsp chopped parsley
- 3 tbsp olive oil

PREPARATION

1. Preheat oven to 180 C (360 F).
2. Cut the tomatoes into wedges and season with garlic, olive oil, salt and pepper.
3. Stir all ingredients together in a pan for a few minutes.
4. Bake for 40 minutes.
5. Make some gaps among the tomatoes and break each egg into it.
6. Cover the baking sheet with foil and bake for another 10 minutes.

Keto Bagels

Difficulty: Easy ¦ Calories 370 ¦ Servings 4
Total Carb: 10 g ¦ Total Fat: 30 g ¦ Protein: 19 g

INGREDIENTS

- 140 g (4.9 oz.) almond flour
- 1 large egg
- 30 g (1 oz.) cream cheese

- 1/5 tsp baking powder
- Shredded mozzarella cheese
- Olive oil

SEASONING MIX

- Poppy seeds
- White sesame seeds

- Minced onion
- Garlic powder

PREPARATION

1. Preheat the oven to 175 C (350 F).
2. Stir all seasoning mix ingredients.
3. Mix part of the seasoning mix, almond flour and baking powder.
4. Add cream cheese and mozzarella cheese. Microwave until all cheese is melted.
5. Add egg and whisk until completely absorbed.
6. Process the mixture with your hands until you obtain a dough.
7. Divide the dough into 4 pieces and shape into bagels.
8. Place the bagels on a greased baking sheet, season with olive oil, salt, and remaining seasoning mix on top.
9. Bake for 20 minutes.

Low-Carb Prawn, Coconut and Tomato Curry

Difficulty: Easy ¦ Calories 335 ¦ Servings 4
Total Carb: 7 g ¦ Total Fat: 26 g ¦ Protein: 19 g

INGREDIENTS

- 350 g (12.3 oz.) prawn
- 200 ml (6.7 oz.) coconut cream
- 200 ml (6.7 oz.) vegetable stock
- 3 tbsp curry paste
- 2 garlic cloves
- 1 tbsp tomato puree
- 1 green chilli
- 1 medium onion
- 2 tbsp vegetable oil
- Coriander springs

PREPARATION

1. Fry the garlic, onion and half the chilli in oil.
2. Add the curry paste and cook for another 2 minutes.
3. Add the stock, coconut cream and tomato puree. Let it simmer for 10 minutes.
4. Add the prawn and cook until they turn opaque.
5. Season with coriander springs and the remaining green chilli.

Keto Cornbread

Difficulty: Easy ¦ Calories 200 ¦ Servings 9
Total Carb: 3.5 g ¦ Total Fat: 18 g ¦ Protein: 7 g

INGREDIENTS

- 170 g (6 oz.) almond flour
- 4 large eggs
- 60 g (2 oz.) confectioners swerve
- 1 tsp baking powder
- 5 tbsp salted butter
- 1 tsp vanilla extract
- Butter and syrup for serving

PREPARATION

1. Preheat the oven to 175 C (350 F), and grease the sides of a baking dish.
2. Mix the almond flour with the baking powder and the sweetener.
3. Mix the eggs, vanilla extract and melted butter in a separate bowl.
4. Combine the two mixtures and beat until well incorporated.
5. When you obtain a thick batter, you can pour it onto your pan. With a spatula, spread the mixture to the edges and corners.
6. Bake for about 25 minutes.
7. Let it cool and then cut into squares. Serve while warm.

Delicious Keto Breakfast Ideas

Keto Banana Bread Muffins

Difficulty: Easy ¦ Calories 210 ¦ Servings 7
Total Carb: 4.5 g ¦ Total Fat: 19 g ¦ Protein: 7 g

INGREDIENTS

- 115 g (4 oz.) almond flour
- 55 g (2 oz.) walnuts (finely chopped)
- 1 large egg
- 40 g (1.4 oz.) sour cream
- ½ tbsp vegetable oil
- ¼ tsp baking soda
- Banana extract
- 55 g (2 oz.) powdered erythritol sweetener

PREPARATION

1. Preheat the oven to 175 C (350 F).
2. Mix all the dry ingredients in a bowl, but don't add the chopped walnuts yet.
3. Beat the egg separately and then add all other wet ingredients. Mix well until smooth.
4. Combine the two mixtures (dry and wet ingredients). Now it is time to add your delicious walnuts!
5. Distribute the mixture among 6 cupcake wrappers. Fill them about 2/3 full, since your mixture will grow up once in the oven.
6. Bake for 20 minutes. Use a toothpick to check when your muffin is ready.
7. Let the banana bread muffins cool before serving.

Keto Coconut Porridge

Difficulty: Easy ¦ Calories 487 ¦ Servings 1
Total Carb: 4 g ¦ Total Fat: 49 g ¦ Protein: 9 g

INGREDIENTS

- 1 egg
- 4 tbsp coconut cream
- 1 pinch ground psyllium husk powder
- 1 tsp coconut flour
- 30 g (1 oz.) butter or coconut oil
- Salt

PREPARATION

1. Mix the egg with the coconut flour, salt and psyllium husk powder.
2. Melt the butter and coconut cream and whisk in the egg mixture.
3. Serve with additional coconut cream, frozen berries or nuts.

Keto Almond Pancakes

Difficulty: Easy ¦ Calories 280 ¦ Servings 2
Total Carb: 6 g ¦ Total Fat: 26 g ¦ Protein: 10 g

INGREDIENTS

- 90 g (3.1 oz.) almond flour
- 2 large egg whites
- 3 tbsp heavy whipping cream
- Confectioners swerve sweetener
- Table salt
- Butter and syrup for serving

PREPARATION

1. Mix all dry ingredients.
2. Stir in the egg whites and the heavy cream and mix well until it is smooth.
3. Pour the mixture over a non-stick pan to form a thick lawyer.
4. Cook both sides of your pancake for 1-2 minutes.
5. Repeat for each pancake.
6. Serve while hot with butter and syrup.

Keto Western Omelette

Difficulty: Easy ¦ Calories 687 ¦ Servings 2
Total Carb: 6 g ¦ Total Fat: 56 g ¦ Protein: 40 g

INGREDIENTS

- 6 eggs
- 75 g (3 oz.) shredded cheese
- 2 tbsp heavy whipping cream
- 150 g (5 oz.) smoked ham
- 50 g (2 oz.) butter
- ½ green bell pepper
- 1 yellow onion
- Salt and pepper

PREPARATION

1. Whisk the eggs and cream until you get a fluffy mixture. Season with salt and pepper.
2. Add half of the cheese.
3. Stir the ham, peppers and onion in frying butter for a few minutes.
4. Add the mix mixture and wait for the omelette to become firm.
5. Sprinkle the rest of the cheese when the omelette is still very hot.

Keto Butter Cookies

Difficulty: Medium ¦ Calories 100 ¦ Servings 10
Total Carb: 2 g ¦ Total Fat: 9 g ¦ Protein: 2 g

INGREDIENTS

- 140 g (5 oz.) almond flour
- 3 tbsp salted butter
- Sliced almonds or shredded coconut (optional)
- ½ tsp vanilla extract
- Powdered erythritol

PREPARATION

1. Preheat oven to 175 C (350 F).
2. Wait until the butter is softened to room temperature and mix all ingredients using hands. You should get a crumbly mixture, which needs to be cohesive.
3. Add sliced almonds or shredded coconut, if required.
4. Form ten balls from your dough and place them on a baking tray prepared with baking paper. Flatten each ball with a fork.
5. Bake for 10 minutes. The cookies must turn golden around edges.

Keto Peanut Butter Cookies

Difficulty: Medium ¦ Calories 100 ¦ Servings 18
Total Carb: 3.5 g ¦ Total Fat: 8 g ¦ Protein: 4 g

INGREDIENTS

- ◆ 260 g (9.2 oz.) salted peanut butter
- ◆ 30 g (1 oz.) almond or coconut flour
- ◆ 1 large egg
- ◆ Powdered erythritol sweetener

PREPARATION

1. Preheat the oven to 175 C (350 F) and line a baking sheet with parchment paper.
2. Combine all ingredients and stir well until you get a thick and dense dough.
3. With your dough, form small balls and place each of them onto the baking sheet.
4. Flatten the balls with your hands or a fork.
5. Bake for 15 minutes.
6. Let it cool until they harden before serving.

Keto Almond Flour Biscuits

Difficulty: Challenging ¦ Calories 350 ¦ Servings 8
Total Carb: 5.5 g ¦ Total Fat: 31 g ¦ Protein: 14 g

INGREDIENTS

- 225 g (8 oz.) almond flour
- 5 slices bacon
- ½ cup heavy whipping cream
- 140 g (5 oz.) shredded cheddar cheese
- 2 tbsp butter (diced)
- Salt

PREPARATION

1. Preheat oven to 175 C (350 F).
2. Cook the bacon and drain it on a paper towel. Let it cool and then cut it into small pieces.
3. Mix almond flour and salt. Add all remaining ingredients (except the bacon) and stir until you get a cohesive dough.
4. Add the bacon and keep stirring.
5. Divide the dough into 8 mounds on a baking sheet.
6. Bake for ½ hour, or until the biscuits are browned.

Low Carb Pumpkin Cheesecake Bars

Difficulty: Challenging ¦ Calories 230 ¦ Servings 24
Total Carb: 4.5 g ¦ Total Fat: 22 g ¦ Protein: 6 g

INGREDIENTS

CRUST

- ◆ 280 g (9.8 oz.) almond flour
- ◆ 6 tbsp salted butter
- ◆ 2 tbsp powdered erythritol sweetener

FILLING

- ◆ 910 g (32 oz.) cream cheese
- ◆ 4 large eggs
- ◆ 225 g (8 oz.) canned pumpkin
- ◆ 1 tsp ground cinnamon
- ◆ ½ tsp ground ginger
- ◆ ½ powdered erythritol sweetener
- ◆ 1/8 tsp ground cloves

CRUST

1. Preheat oven to 175 C (350 F), and line the bottom and the sides of a baking dish with parchment paper.
2. Melt the butter and combine it with erythritol. Add the almond flour and keep stirring.
3. Transfer the butter mixture to the baking dish, and form a flare crust.
4. Bake it for 15 minutes.

FILLING

1. Mix the cream cheese and the erythritol with a hand mixer.
2. Add eggs, one at a time, and beat the mixture until well combined. It should be airy and fluffy.
3. Pour half of the mixture over the crust and spread it evenly. This will be the first layer of your cheesecake.
4. Add the remaining ingredients to the rest of your mixture and mix well.
5. Build additional layers over the cheesecake crust with your mixture.
6. Bake for about 1 hour.
7. Let it cool and then refrigerate overnight before cutting and serving it.
8.

Mushroom Hash with Poached Eggs

Difficulty: Easy ¦ Calories: 283 ¦ Serves: 4
Carbs: 15 g ¦ Fat: 17 g ¦ Protein: 15 g

INGREDIENTS

- 500 g mushrooms, quartered
- 4 large eggs
- 500 g fresh tomatoes, chopped
- 4 tsp seed mix
- 2 large onions, halved and sliced
- 1 tsp smoked paprika
- 1 ½ tbsp rapeseed oil
- 1 tbsp fresh thyme leaves
- Extra thyme leaves, to garnish

PREPARATION

1. Heat the oil in a pan and stir fry the onions. Cover with a lid to leave the onions to cook in their own steam.

2. Add in the mushrooms and the thyme and cook for 5 minutes, or until softened.

3. Stir in the tomatoes and the smoked paprika. Cover with a lid and cook for 5 minutes.

4. Stir in the seed mix.

5. Poach the eggs in lightly simmering water.

6. Serve the eggs on top of the mushroom hash, with additional thyme.

Scrambled Eggs with Basil, Spinach & Tomatoes

Difficulty: Easy ¦ Calories: 297 ¦ Serves: 2
Carbs: 10 g ¦ Fat: 17 g ¦ Protein: 20 g

INGREDIENTS

- 4 large eggs
- 3 tomatoes, halved
- 175 g baby spinach
- 1/3 small pack basil, chopped
- 1 tbsp + 1 tsp rapeseed oil
- 4 tbsp natural yoghurt

PREPARATION

1. Heat 1 tsp oil in a pan and stir fry the tomatoes over medium heat.
2. Meanwhile, beat the eggs in a bowl with 2 tbsp water, the yoghurt, basil, and black pepper.
3. Transfer the tomatoes to your serving plates. In the same pan, cook the spinach for a few minutes.
4. Heat the remaining oil and pour in the egg mixture, making scrambled eggs.
5. Add the spinach and the scrambled eggs into your serving plates.

Keto Mushroom Brunch

Difficulty: Easy ¦ Calories: 154 ¦ Serves: 4
Carbs: 1 g ¦ Fat: 11 g ¦ Protein: 13 g

INGREDIENTS

- 250 g mushrooms, sliced
- 160 g kale
- 4 medium egg
- 1 garlic clove, crushed
- 1 tbsp extra virgin olive oil

PREPARATION

1. Heat the oil in a pan and fry the garlic for 1-2 minutes. Add in the mushrooms and cook for a few minutes, or until soft. Stir in the kale.

2. Season with salt and pepper to taste.

3. Crack in the eggs and cook for 2-3 minutes. Cover the pan with a lid and cook for further 2-3 minutes.

Keto Mushrooms Baked Eggs with Squashed Tomatoes

Difficulty: Easy ¦ Calories: 147 ¦ Serves: 2
Carbs: 5 g ¦ Fat: 8 g ¦ Protein: 12 g

INGREDIENTS

- 2 large flat mushrooms, chopped
- 2 large eggs
- 2 tomatoes, halved
- ½ garlic clove, grated
- 2 handfuls rocket
- 1 tbsp rapeseed oil
- 1 few thyme leaves

PREPARATION

1. Heat oven to 200 C.

2. Brush the mushrooms with the oil and garlic, then place into two greased gratin dishes. Season with salt and pepper.

3. Top with chopped stalks and thyme. Cover with foil and bake for 20-25 minutes.

4. Once ready, remove the foil. Add the tomatoes and break an egg onto each mushroom.

5. Return to oven for 10 minutes.

6. Top with the rocket before serving.

Keto Tomato Baked Eggs

Difficulty: Easy ¦ Calories: 204 ¦ Serves: 4
Carbs: 7 g ¦ Fat: 16 g ¦ Protein: 9 g

INGREDIENTS

- 900 g ripe vine tomatoes, cut into wedges
- 3 tbsp olive oil
- 3 garlic cloves, peeled and sliced
- 4 large eggs
- 2 tbsp chopped parsley

PREPARATION

1. Preheat the oven to 180 C.
2. Spread the tomato wedges over an ovenproof dish. Sprinkle with the garlic and drizzle with the oil. Season to taste.
3. Stir well and bake for 40 minutes.
4. Make four gaps among your tomatoes and break an egg into each space.
5. Return to oven for 10 minutes.
6. Scatter with herbs before serving.

Keto Green Eggs

Difficulty: Easy ¦ Calories: 298 ¦ Serves: 2
Carbs: 8 g ¦ Fat: 20 g ¦ Protein: 18 g

INGREDIENTS

- 2 large eggs
- 200 g spinach
- 2 garlic cloves, sliced
- 2 tbsp Greek yoghurt
- 2 trimmed leeks, sliced
- ½ tsp fennel seeds
- ½ tsp coriander seeds
- 1 ½ tbsp rapeseed oil
- The juice of 1 lemon
- Chilli flakes

PREPARATION

1. Heat the rapeseed oil in a frying pan. Stir fry the leeks until soft. Season with salt.

2. Add in the coriander, garlic, fennel and chilli flakes.

3. After a couple of minutes, add in the spinach. Keep cooking everything on low heat until the spinach has wilted. Set aside.

4. Add extra oil into the pan and crack in the eggs. Cook until well fried.

5. Stir the yoghurt in the spinach mix. Transfer to your serving plates and top with the fried egg.

6. Season with the lemon juice, salt, black pepper and chilli flakes.

Bacon & Avocado Frittata

Difficulty: Easy ¦ Calories: 467 ¦ Serves: 4
Carbs: 7 g ¦ Fat: 38 g ¦ Protein: 22 g

INGREDIENTS

- 6 eggs, beaten
- 200 g mixed salad leaves
- 1 large avocado, halved, stoned, and cut into chunks
- 12 baby plum tomatoes, halved
- 3 tbsp olive oil
- 8 smoked bacon slices
- 2 tsp red wine vinegar
- 1 small red chilli, chopped

PREPARATION

1. Heat an ovenproof pan and fry the bacon. Chop into large pieces and set aside. Use some kitchen paper to absorb excess fat, if needed.

2. Heat 1 tbsp oil in a pan. In a bowl, break the eggs and add ½ of the bacon, and season with salt. Cook on low heat in the pan.

3. Place the avocado slices and the remaining bacon. Grill for 4-5 minutes.

4. Mix the chilli, vinegar and remaining oil and use this mixture to season the frittata.

5. Serve with the salad leaves and tomatoes.

Prawn and Herb Omelette

Difficulty: Easy ¦ Calories: 288 ¦ Serves: 2
Carbs: 19 g ¦ Fat: 21 g ¦ Protein: 6 g

INGREDIENTS

- 4 eggs
- 250 ml milk
- 350 g prawns, cooked, peeled, chopped
- 60 g butter, diced
- 1 ½ cups mixed herbs

- 2 spring onions, sliced
- 1 cucumber, sliced
- 1 fennel, sliced
- Toasted sesame seeds, to serve
- Toasted nori sheets, cut into squares

LEMON-TAHINI DRESSING

- 1 tbsp tahini
- 2 tbsp extra virgin olive oil
- 2 tbsp honey

- 2 tbsp chopped chives
- 1 lemon cut into wedges, to serve

PREPARATION

1. To make the dressing, mix the tahini, olive oil, honey, lemon juice and 1 tbsp water. season with salt and stir in the chives.

2. In another bowl, mix the milk, herbs and eggs.

3. Melt ½ butter in a non-stick frying pan, then add in the egg mixture. Use a spatula to draw the cooked egg towards the centre of the pan, without breaking them up.

4. Add in half the prawn and cook until they are warmed. Transfer to a serving plate and repeat with remaining ingredients.

5. Serve topped with fennel, cucumber, spring onion, sesame seeds and nori, and the dressing.

Mexican Egg Roll

Difficulty: Easy ¦ Calories: 133 ¦ Serves: 2
Carbs: 2 g ¦ Fat: 10 g ¦ Protein: 9 g

INGREDIENTS

- 1 large egg
- 2 tbsp tomato salsa
- 1 tbsp rapeseed oil
- 1 tbsp fresh coriander

PREPARATION

1. Beat the egg along with 1 tbsp water.

2. Heat the oil in a pan and add the egg. Swirl around the base of the frying pan until you get a pancake, and cook until set.

3. Remove from heat and spread the tomato salsa over the pancake. Sprinkle with the coriander and roll it up.

Keto Healthy Meals

Keto Oven Baked Chicken Breasts

Difficulty: Easy ¦ Calories 480 ¦ Servings 2
Total Carb: 9 g ¦ Total Fat: 22 g ¦ Protein: 57 g

INGREDIENTS

- 2 boneless chicken breasts
- 85 g (3 oz.) cream cheese
- 85 g (3 oz.) fresh spinach leaves (chopped)
- Sun-dried tomatoes (chopped)
- Salt and pepper
- Garlic powder

PREPARATION

1. Preheat the oven to 200 C (400 F).
2. Slice each chicken breast in half. If the meat is too moist, you can pat it dry with paper towels.
3. Spread the chicken breasts on a baking tray lined with parchment paper. Add garlic powder, and salt and pepper.
4. Microwave the cream cheese until very soft. Meanwhile, cook the spinach leaves.
5. Stir together the cream cheese and the spinach in a bowl.
6. Spread the mixture across your chicken breasts and then bake for 20 minutes.

Keto Super-Easy Stir Fry

Difficulty: Easy ¦ Calories 400 ¦ Servings 4
Total Carb: 16 g ¦ Total Fat: 40 g ¦ Protein: 56 g

INGREDIENTS

- 700 g (24.7 oz.) boneless chicken thighs
- 300 g (10.5 oz.) broccoli florets
- 5 shiitake mushrooms (sliced)
- 1 carrot (cut into pieces)

CAULIFLOWER RICE

- 1 kg (35 oz.) cauliflower florets
- 2 tbsp coconut oil
- Salt and pepper

- 4 spring onions
- 3 tbsp coconut oil, for frying
- 2 baby bok choy
- Stir fry sauce

PREPARATION

1. Fry the chicken thighs in coconut oil and then transfer to a plate.
2. In the same pan, stir-fry the spring onion with the other vegetables.
3. Return the chick to the pan, pour some stir-fry sauce and mix all the ingredients.
4. Season with salt and pepper, or your choice of spices.
5. To make the cauliflower rice, you should start by processing the cauliflower florets in a food processor.
6. Stir-fry the florets in coconut oil and then serve with your choice of vegetables and sauces.

Keto Chicken Salad with Avocado and Bacon

Difficulty: Easy ¦ Calories 640 ¦ Servings 2
Total Carb: 9 g ¦ Total Fat: 38 g ¦ Protein: 57 g

INGREDIENTS

- 115 g (4 oz.) cooked chicken
- 1 large avocado
- 5 slices bacon (crumbled)
- Shredded cheddar cheese.
- Diced celery
- Scallions (thinly sliced)
- Salt and pepper
- Caesar dressing or your choice of dressing

PREPARATION

1. Chop the chicken pieces and cook the bacon.
2. Mix all ingredients in a large salad bowl.
3. Season with salt and pepper and add your choice of dressing.

Keto Chicken Garam Masala

Difficulty: Easy ┊ Calories 643 ┊ Servings 4
Total Carb: 6 g ┊ Total Fat: 51 g ┊ Protein: 39 g

INGREDIENTS

CHICKEN

- 650 g (1 ½ lbs) chicken breast
- 300 ml (1 ¼ cups) unsweetened coconut cream
- 1 red bell pepper
- 1 tbsp fresh parsley
- 3 tbsp butter
- Salt

GARAM MASALA

- 1 tsp chilli powder
- 1 tsp turmeric
- 1 tsp ground cardamom
- 1 tsp paprika powder
- 1 tsp coriander seed
- 1 tsp ground cumin
- 1 pinch ground nutmeg

PREPARATION

1. Preheat oven to 175 C (350 F).
2. Mix all the spices for the garam masala.
3. Cut the chicken breasts and fry in butter over medium-high heat.
4. Add half of the garam masala mix and stir well.
5. Place the chicken in a baking dish and season with salt.
6. Mix the bell pepper (finely sliced) with the coconut cream and the remaining spices mixture.
7. Pour the coconut cream mixture over the chicken and bake for 20 minutes.
8. Garnish with finely chopped fresh parsley before serving.

Low-Carb Pork Shoulder Chops with Cauliflower Au Gratin

Difficulty: Easy ¦ Calories 813 ¦ Servings 6
Total Carb: 9 g ¦ Total Fat: 64 g ¦ Protein: 47 g

INGREDIENTS

- 900 g (30 oz.) pork shoulder chops
- 900 g (30 oz.) cauliflower florets
- 150 g (5 1/3 oz.) bacon
- 150 ml (2/3 cup) heavy whipping cream
- 200 g (7 oz.) cream cheese
- 75 g (3 oz.) leeks
- 200 g (7 oz.) shredded cheese
- 200 g (7 oz.) shredded cheddar cheese
- 1 garlic clove
- Salt and pepper

PREPARATION

1. Preheat oven to 200 C (400 F)
2. Boil the cauliflower florets and then let them drain aside.
3. Dice the bacon and fry in butter.
4. Mix the cream, cream cheese and part of the grated cheese in a bowl.
5. Finely chop the leeks and add to the cheese mixture.
6. Add the cauliflower and bacon.
7. Season with salt, pepper and spices.
8. Bake for ½ hour.
9. Meanwhile, cook the pork chops either in a pan or grilled.

Low Carb Bacon Tenderloin with Roasted Garlic Mash

Difficulty: Easy ¦ Calories 1040 ¦ Servings 4
Total Carb: 13 g ¦ Total Fat: 88 g ¦ Protein: 49 g

INGREDIENTS

BACON-WRAPPED PORK TENDERLOIN

- 650 g (1 ½ lbs) pork tenderloin
- 150 g (5 oz.) cream cheese
- 200 g (7 oz.) bacon
- 30 g (1 oz.) sun-dried tomatoes
- 175 ml (3/4 cup) heavy whipping cream
- Olive oil
- Butter
- 1 garlic clove
- 2 tbsp fresh sage

ROASTED GARLIC CAULIFLOWER MASH

- 450 g (1 lb) cauliflower
- 110 g (4 oz.) butter
- 1 whole garlic
- 1 tbsp olive oil
- Salt and pepper

1. Make the cauliflower mash by trimming the cauliflower and cutting it into small florets.

2. Boil the cauliflower and let it drain.

3. Roast the carling into the oven, then place it with the cauliflower and some butter in a food processor. Mix until smooth.

4. Preheat the oven to 175 C (350 F).

5. Mix sun-dried tomatoes, garlic, cream cheese and sage in a small bowl.

6. Season the pork tenderloin with salt and pepper and cut it to make a pocket.

7. Add half of the cream cheese mixture in the pork and use the bacon slices to wrap and seal.

8. Bake the pork in the oven for 20 minutes.

9. Leave the meat to rest. Meanwhile, pour the juices from the baking dish in a pan and add the remaining heavy cream and the rest of the filling. Let the ingredients simmer for a few minutes.

10. Slice the pork diagonally and serve with the cauliflower mash and the filling sauce.

Keto Hamburger Patties with Creamy Tomato Sauce and Fried Cabbage

Difficulty: Medium ¦ Calories 923 ¦ Servings 4
Total Carb: 10 g ¦ Total Fat: 78 g ¦ Protein: 42 g

INGREDIENTS

HAMBURGER PATTIES

- 650 g (1 ½ lbs) ground beef
- 75 g (3 oz.) feta cheese
- 1 medium egg
- Fresh parsley (finely chopped)
- Olive oil and butter, for frying
- Salt and pepper

GRAVY

- 175 ml (3/4 cup) heavy whipping cream
- 2 tbsp tomato paste
- Fresh parsley

FRIED CABBAGE

- 650 g (1 ½ lbs) shredded green cabbage
- Salt and pepper
- 125 g (4 ½ oz.) butter

PREPARATION

1. Mix all the patties hamburgers in a large bowl with your hands or a wooden spoon.

2. With wet hands, form your patties.

3. Fry patties with butter and olive oil for at least 10 minutes.

4. Whisk all the gravy ingredients in another bowl.

5. Add the gravy mixture to the pan and stir for a few minutes.

6. Keep the patties warm. Meanwhile, shred the cabbage and fry it in a pan with some butter.

7. Season with salt and pepper the hamburger patties and the cabbage and serve together.

Keto Turkey Burgers with Tomato Butter

Difficulty: Medium ¦ Calories 834 ¦ Servings 4
Total Carb: 8 g ¦ Total Fat: 75 g ¦ Protein: 33 g

INGREDIENTS

TURKEY PATTIES

- 650 g (1 ½ lbs) ground turkey
- 650 g (1 ½ lbs) green cabbage
- ½ yellow onion
- 75 g (2 oz.) butter
- 1 medium egg
- 1 tsp crushed coriander seed or dried thyme
- Salt and pepper

TOMATO BUTTER

- 110 g (3 oz.) butter
- 1 tsp red wine vinegar
- 1 tbsp tomato paste

PREPARATION

1. Preheat oven to 100 C (220 F).
2. Mix all the patties ingredients and shape your patties with wet hands.
3. Fry the patties in butter and keep them warm in the oven.
4. Meanwhile, you can prepare your sides. First, shred the cabbage and fry it in butter. Season with salt and pepper.
5. Whip all the tomato butter ingredients together in a bowl with an electric hand mixer.
6. Serve the patties, the cabbage and the tomato butter together.

Keto Chicken with Lemon and Butter

Difficulty: Medium ¦ Calories 984 ¦ Servings 4
Total Carb: 0.3 g ¦ Total Fat: 82 g ¦ Protein: 58 g

INGREDIENTS

- 1.5 kg (3 lbs) chicken
- 150 g (5 oz.) butter
- 2 tsp barbecue seasoning
- 2 yellow onions
- 1 lemon
- 60 ml (1/4 cup) water
- Salt and pepper

PREPARATION

1. Preheat the oven to 175 C (350 F).
2. Season the chicken with salt and pepper. For extra taste, rub the meat with the barbecue seasoning, then place it in a greased baking dish.
3. Add the onions, cut into wedges, and some lemon slices in the baking dish, too.
4. Slice the butter and place it on top of the chicken.
5. Back the chicken for 1 ½ hour. It may take more, depending on the size of the meat. Don't forget to add water, if necessary, to keep the meat juicy.

Perfect Keto-Friendly Soups

Thai Chicken Coconut Soup

Difficulty: Easy ¦ Calories: 211 ¦ Serves: 4
Carbs: 16 g ¦ Fat: 24 g ¦ Protein: 11 g

INGREDIENTS

- 300 ml chicken broth
- 450 g boneless, skinless chicken thighs, cut into pieces
- 115 g shiitake mushrooms, chopped
- 1 tbsp fish sauce
- 1 can coconut milk
- 1 tbsp freshly minced ginger
- 1 tbsp extra virgin olive oil
- The juice of 1 lime
- Cilantro leaves, to garnish
- Chilli oil, to garnish (optional)

PREPARATION

1. Heat the oil in a pan over medium heat. Stir fry the ginger for 1 minute, then add in the mushrooms and cook for 5 minutes.

2. Add coconut milk, fish sauce, and broth. Bring to the boil. Add the chicken and leave to simmer for 15 minutes, or until it is no longer pink.

3. Turn the heat off. Stir in the lime juice.

4. Serve the chicken soup garnished with cilantro and chilli oil (optional).

Keto-friendly Cauliflower Soup

Difficulty: Easy ¦ Calories: 176 ¦ Serves: 4-6
Carbs: 14 g ¦ Fat: 38 g ¦ Protein: 8 g

INGREDIENTS

- 1 large cauliflower, cut into florets
- 850 ml vegetable stock
- 100 ml single cream
- 1 garlic clove, crushed
- 1 celery stick, chopped
- 4 thyme sprigs
- 1 onion, chopped
- 2 tbsp olive oil
- ½ tbsp ground cumin
- ½ small bunch of parsley, chopped

PREPARATION

1. Heat the oven to 200 C.
2. Spread the cauliflower florets in a roasting tin and drizzle with 1 tbsp olive oil, thyme and cumin. Roast for 15 minutes. Discard the thyme once ready.
3. Heat the remaining oil in a saucepan and fry the onion and celery over medium heat for 10 minutes, or until softened. Add in the garlic and ¾ of the cauliflower. Add the stock and bring to a simmer. Cook for 10-12 minutes.
4. With a food processor, pulse the cauliflower mixture until smooth.
5. Season to taste and serve with the reserved cauliflower, parsley, and extra olive oil.

Broccoli Cheddar Soup

Difficulty: Easy ¦ Calories: 231 ¦ Serves: 4
Carbs: 11 g ¦ Fat: 18 g ¦ Protein: 5 g

INGREDIENTS

- 1 small onion, diced
- 2 small heads broccoli, cut into florets plus the stems cut into pieces
- 85 g cheddar, grated
- 3 tbsp all-purpose flour
- 60 ml half-and-half
- 120 ml vegetable broth
- 3 tbsp unsalted butter
- 1 pinch of nutmeg
- 2 cloves garlic, crushed
- Greek full-fat yoghurt or sour cream, to garnish

PREPARATION

1. Melt the butter in a medium pot over medium heat. Cook the onion for 5 minutes, then stir in the garlic and cook until fragrant. Add the flour and stir constantly for 3 minutes, or until it turns golden.

2. Add the half-and-half and the broth and bring to the boil. Reduce the heat and stir in the broccoli. Save a few pieces of broccoli for garnish. Leave to simmer for 15 minutes, or until broccoli is tender.

3. With an immersion blender, puree the soup in the pot.

4. Whisk in the cheddar and season to taste. Add the nutmeg.

5. Garnish with extra broccoli, Greek yoghurt or sour cream.

Keto Main Meals

Cauliflower Steaks with Roasted Red Pepper and Olive Salsa

Difficulty: Easy ¦ Calories: 277 ¦ Serves: 2
Carbs: 11 g ¦ Fat: 21 g ¦ Protein: 9 g

INGREDIENTS

- 1 big cauliflower
- 4 black olives, pitted
- 1 roasted red pepper
- 2 tbsp olive oil
- 1 tsp capers

- 2 tbsp toasted flaked almonds
- ½ tbsp red wine vinegar
- ½ tsp smoked paprika
- 1 small handful parsley

PREPARATION

1. Preheat the oven to 200 C and prepare a baking tray.

2. Slice the cauliflower into two steaks, and save some florets for later.

3. Rub the paprika and ½ tbsp oil over the steaks and season with salt. Place onto the trash and roast for 20 minutes.

4. To make the salsa, chop the parsley, olives, peppers, and capers. Mix in a bowl and season to taste.

5. Serve the cauliflower steaks topped with salsa and flaked almonds.

Steak with Porcini Butter and Charred Onion

Difficulty: Easy ¦ Calories: 279 ¦ Serves: 4
Carbs: 19 g ¦ Fat: 13 g ¦ Protein: 23 g

INGREDIENTS

- 4 x 150 g minute steaks
- 100 g unsalted butter, softened
- 2 tbsp dried porcini mushrooms, chopped
- 1 bunch salad onions

- 2 garlic cloves, crushed
- 2 lemons, halved
- 2 tbsp thyme leaves
- 1 tbsp extra virgin olive oil

PREPARATION

1. Immerse the porcini in a bowl with boiling water. Once the liquid is absorbed, add garlic, thyme and butter. Season with salt and spread half of this butter over the steaks.

2. Cook the steaks for 1-2 minutes on each side until medium-rare, or cook to your liking.

3. Cover the steaks with foil and leave to rest.

4. Meanwhile, brush the onions and the lemons with olive oil and fry for 2 minutes in a hot pan.

5. Serve the steaks with lemon and onion, and the remaining mushrooms butter.

Keto Japanese Kingfish Lettuce Cups

Difficulty: Easy ¦ Calories: 275 ¦ Serves: 4
Carbs: 15 g ¦ Fat: 21 g ¦ Protein: 32 g

INGREDIENTS

- 800 g kingfish fillet, skin off, cut into pieces
- 2 little gem lettuces, leaves separated, shredded
- ¼ red cabbage, shredded
- 4 watermelon radishes, sliced
- 6 spring onions, sliced
- 2 tbsp light soy sauce
- 2 tbsp oyster sauce
- 2 tbsp peanut oil
- 1 garlic clove, crushed
- 1 tbsp fish sauce
- Your choice of sauce, to serve

PREPARATION

1. Place the kingfish fillet in a food processor and pulse until it is finely chopped.
2. In a frying pan, high the oil and fry the onion and garlic. After 2 minutes, add the fish and cook until starting to colour.
3. Add the soy sauce, fish sauce and oyster sauce. Leave to cook until the sauces have reduced.
4. Serve this mixture in lettuce leaves. Top with radish slices, cabbage and your choice of sauce.

Chicken Salad Stuffed Avocado

Difficulty: Easy ¦ Calories: 431 ¦ Serves: 4
Carbs: 11 g ¦ Fat: 30 g ¦ Protein: 31 g

INGREDIENTS

- 2 avocados, pitted
- 2 tbsp Greek yoghurt
- The juice of 1 lemon
- 150 g shredded cooked chicken
- 30 g mayonnaise
- 1 ½ tsp Dijon mustard
- ½ red onion, minced
- Chopped parsley, to garnish

PREPARATION

1. Scoop out avocados, but make sure to leave a small border. Dice the avocado flesh.

2. To make the chicken salad, mix the meat, onion, yoghurt, mayo, mustard and lemon juice in a bowl. Add in the diced avocado and season with salt and pepper to taste.

3. Serve the salad into the 4 avocado halves, and garnish with chopped parsley.

Keto Cauliflower Chowder

Difficulty: Easy ¦ Calories: 288 ¦ Serves: 6-8
Carbs: 12 g ¦ Fat: 16 g ¦ Protein: 15 g

INGREDIENTS

- 4 slices bacon, cut into pieces
- 2 medium carrots, peeled and chopped
- 1 l vegetable broth
- 1 medium yellow onion, chopped
- 1 head cauliflower, cut into florets
- 2 stalk celery, chopped
- 2 cloves garlic, minced
- 2 tbsp flour
- 2 sprigs thyme, chopped
- 60 ml whole milk

PREPARATION

1. Cook the bacon in a large pot until crispy. Transfer to a plate lined with a paper towel and drain part of the excess fat.

2. In the same pot, cook the celery, carrots and onion. Season to taste. Add in the garlic and the flour and stir well for 2 minutes. Add cauliflower and thyme.

3. Pour in the milk and vegetable broth and bring to a boil. Reduce heat and leave to simmer for 15 minutes.

4. Garnish with bacon and season to taste.

Low-Carb Pumpkin Spaghetti

Difficulty: Easy ¦ Calories: 144 ¦ Serves: 4
Carbs: 4 g ¦ Fat: 12 g ¦ Protein: 22 g

INGREDIENTS

- 1 butternut pumpkin, halved, seeds removed
- 2 garlic cloves, sliced
- 1 bunch sage, leaves picked
- 4 sliced ham, torn into pieces
- 60 g butter, chopped
- 55 g almonds, chopped
- Extra almonds, to serve
- Your choice of sauce

PREPARATION

1. Preheat the oven to 250 C.
2. With a mandolin or a spiraliser, turn your pumpkin into spaghetti.
3. Spread the sage leaves, ham, almonds and garlic onto a roasting pan. Scatter butter.
4. Add in the pumpkin spaghetti and bake for 10-15 minutes.
5. Top with extra almonds and serve with your choice of keto-friendly sauce.

Keto Chili

Difficulty: Medium ¦ Calories: 435 ¦ Serves: 8
Carbs: 11g ¦ Fat: 33 g ¦ Protein: 25 g

INGREDIENTS

- 1 kg ground beef
- 3 slices bacon, cut into strips
- 1 green bell pepper, chopped
- 2 celery stalks, chopped
- ¼ medium yellow onion, chopped
- 2 cloves garlic, minced
- 2 tbsp smoked paprika
- 2 tsp dried oregano
- 2 tbsp chilli powder
- 2 tsp ground cumin
- 300 ml beef broth
- 60 g mushrooms, sliced
- Shredded cheddar, to garnish
- Sour cream, to garnish
- Sliced avocado, to garnish
- Sliced green onions, to garnish

PREPARATION

1. Cook the bacon in a pot over medium heat. Remove from heat once crispy.
2. In the same pot, cook the pepper, celery, onion, and mushrooms. Add the garlic and cook until fragrant.
3. Add the beef and cook well.
4. Stir in the cumin, oregano, chilli powder and paprika. Season to taste.
5. Add the broth and bring to a simmer, then cook for 15 minutes.
6. Serve into bowls, topped with sour cream, cheese, avocado and green onions.

Spinach & Ricotta Gnocchi

Difficulty: Medium ¦ Calories: 287 ¦ Serves: 4
Carbs: 19 g ¦ Fat: 15 g ¦ Protein: 20 g

INGREDIENTS

- 200 g spinach, washed
- 2 eggs
- 85 g plain flour
- 140 g ricotta
- 1 garlic clove, crushed
- 1 small handful parsley leaves, chopped
- 100 g parmesan (or any vegetarian alternative)
- Freshly grated nutmeg
- Olive oil, to serve
- Rocket, to serve

PREPARATION

1. Place the spinach in a bowl in boiling water. Leave for 2 minutes, then drain and allow to cool. Remove extra liquid with a clean tea towel.

2. In a large bowl, mix the spinach, eggs, ricotta, parsley, garlic, cheese and nutmeg. Season with salt and pepper. With a fork, stir thoroughly until everything is perfectly mixed. With wed hands, form the egg mixture into balls. Refrigerate for at least ½ hour.

3. Once ready to cook, bring a pan of water to the boil.

4. Cook the gnocchi for about 1-2 minutes.

5. Serve the gnocchi drizzled with olive oil, rocket and extra cheese.

Keto-friendly Crustless Quiche

Difficulty: Medium ¦ Calories: 401 ¦ Serves: 6
Carbs: 3 g ¦ Fat: 34 g ¦ Protein: 19 g

INGREDIENTS

- 100 g chopped pancetta (or smoked bacon)
- 200 g asparagus, trimmed (or broccoli)
- 20 g butter
- 150 g double cream
- 80 g parmesan cheese (or gruyere)
- 8 large eggs
- 1 onion, chopped

PREPARATION

1. Heat oven to 180 C and prepare a cake tin.
2. Melt the butter in a pan. Add in the pancetta and onion and cook for 10 minutes.
3. Bring a pan of salted water to the boil to cook the asparagus (or the broccoli).
4. In a bowl, whisk the cream, eggs and 2/3 of the cheese. Season with salt and pepper. Add in the onion and bacon.
5. Pour the mixture into the tip. Top with the vegetables and sprinkle the remaining cheese. Bake for ½ hour.

Keto West Indian Spiced Aubergine Curry

Difficulty: Medium ¦ Calories: 157 ¦ Serves: 2
Carbs: 13 g ¦ Fat: 9 g ¦ Protein: 4 g

INGREDIENTS

- 1 large aubergine
- 2 tbsp tomato puree
- 3 spring onions, chopped
- 1 tsp ground coriander
- 1 tsp ground cumin
- 1 cm piece of ginger, peeled and chopped
- 1 ½ tbsp rapeseed oil

- 2 tsp caster sugar
- ½ tsp ground turmeric
- ½ bunch coriander, shredded
- ½ green chilli, chopped
- Cooked cauliflower rice, to serve
- Natural full-fat yoghurt, to serve
- Lime wedges, to serve

PREPARATION

1. Mix all the dry spices with 1 tsp salt in a bowl.
2. Slice the aubergine and score both sides with the tip of a knife. Rub with the spice mix.
3. In a bowl, put 150 ml water, chilli, tomato puree, sugar and ginger.
4. Heat the oil in a pan and cook the aubergine for 5 minutes on each side. Add the tomato puree mix and cook for 15-20 minutes. Add more water if necessary. Season to taste.
5. Serve the aubergine scattered over with spring onions and coriander. Serve with cauliflower rice, yoghurt and lime wedges.

Low-Carb Cauliflower Pizza

Difficulty: Medium ¦ Calories: 354 ¦ Serves: 1 pizza
Carbs: 18 g ¦ Fat: 15 g ¦ Protein: 13 g

INGREDIENTS

- 60 ml tomato pasta sauce
- 100 g mozzarella, thinly sliced
- 60 ml pesto
- 250 mixed cherry tomatoes, halved
- Baby basil leaves, to garnish

CAULIFLOWER DOUGH

- 1 big cauliflower
- 30 g grated parmesan
- 75 g almonds
- 2 eggs
- 1 tbsp olive oil

PREPARATION

1. Preheat the oven to 140 C and prepare two baking trays with baking paper.

2. Chop the cauliflower and use a food processor to pulse until it is finely chopped. Using a clean cloth, squeeze and remove all the excess liquid and moisture.

3. Spread the cauliflower over the trays and bake for 15 minutes. Once completely dried out, leave to cool.

4. Return the cauliflower to the food processor and add the almonds, parmesan, and the eggs. Season with salt and pepper. Process until you get a smooth dough.

5. Spread the cauliflower mixture to the baking tray. Increase oven to 180 C and roast for 25/30 minutes, or until golden.

6. Increase the oven once again to 250 C. Spread the pesto and tomato sauce over the cauliflower base and top with mozzarella. Roast for additional 10 minutes, or until the cheese is melted.

7. Garnish with basil leaves and serve your delicious pizza.

Keto Ginger Chicken Stir-Fry

Difficulty: Medium ¦ Calories: 411 ¦ Serves: 4
Carbs: 15 g ¦ Fat: 39 g ¦ Protein: 24 g

INGREDIENTS

- 700 g boneless chicken thighs, cut into pieces
- 300 g broccoli, cut into florets
- 4 spring onions, cut into batons

STIR-FRY SAUCE

- 6 cm piece of ginger, cut into matchsticks
- 4 garlic cloves, chopped
- 1 tbsp coconut oil
- 250 ml chicken broth
- 1 long red chilli, cut into matchsticks

CAULIFLOWER RICE

- 1 head cauliflower
- 2 tbsp coconut oil
- Salt and pepper

- 5 shiitake mushrooms, sliced
- 2 baby bok choy, chopped
- 1 carrot, cut into matchsticks
- 3 tbsp coconut oil

- 2 tbsp toasted sesame oil
- 1 tbsp coconut sugar
- 3 tbsp tamari
- 2 tsp sesame seeds
- 2 tsp tapioca flour

1. To make the stir-fry sauce, heat the coconut oil over medium heat. Add in the garlic, chilli and ginger. Cook for 1 minute. Pour in the tamari and chicken broth, coconut sugar, pepper, and sesame seeds. Bring to a simmer. Add in the tapioca mixture and bring to the boil. Once ready, set aside.

2. Melt 1 tbsp coconut oil in a wok and stir fry the chicken for 5 minutes. Transfer to a plate.

3. Stir fry the spring onion in the remaining coconut oil. Add the other vegetables and cook for 5 minutes.

4. Return the chicken to the pan, pour in the stir fry sauce, and cook everything together for 2 minutes. Season with salt and pepper, if needed.

5. To make the cauliflower rice, place the florets in a food processor and pulse until you get a fine rice-like texture. Heat the coconut oil and stir fry the cauliflower rice for a few minutes. Season with salt and pepper.

6. Serve the cauliflower rice topped with the stir fry mixture, extra sesame seeds and coriander leaves.

Healthy and Indulgent Keto Salads

Keto Cobb Egg Salad

Difficulty: Easy ¦ Calories: 217 ¦ Serves: 6
Carbs: 8 g ¦ Fat: 16 g ¦ Protein: 29 g

INGREDIENTS

- 8 hard-boiled eggs, cut into eight pieces
- 1 avocado, sliced
- 8 strips bacon, crumbled
- 2 tbsp red wine vinegar
- 3 tbsp Greek full-fat yoghurt

- 3 tbsp mayonnaise
- 2 tbsp freshly chopped chives
- 50 g blue cheese, crumbled (plus extra to garnish)
- 8-10 cherry tomatoes, halved

PREPARATION

1. Mix the mayonnaise, red wine vinegar and yoghurt in a bowl. Season with salt and pepper.
2. In another bowl, mix the eggs, avocado, bacon, blue cheese and tomatoes.
3. Gently fold the mayonnaise dressing into the eggs bowl.
4. Garnish with chives, extra cheese, and your choice of toppings, or extra tomatoes.

Keto Red-Braised Pork Belly with Apple Salad

Difficulty: Easy ¦ Calories: 234 ¦ Serves: 4
Carbs: 21 g ¦ Fat: 19 g ¦ Protein: 27 g

INGREDIENTS

- 1.2 kg boneless pork belly, cut into pieces
- 250 ml light soy sauce
- 500 ml dark soy sauce
- 10 cm piece of ginger, sliced
- 1 bunch spring onions
- 10 star anise
- 1 kg caster sugar
- 3 cinnamon quills
- 2 Granny Smith apples, cut into matchsticks
- The juice of 1 lemon
- 1 bunch coriander, leaves picked
- 2 tbsp olive oil

PREPARATION

1. Place the pork belly, skin-side up, in a dish and sprinkle with salt. Refrigerate for 2 hours.

2. Mix the sugar, ginger, spices, green spring onions, and soy sauces in a stockpot. Cover with water and leave to simmer until the sugar dissolves. Cover with a lid and leave to simmer for at least 1 hour.

3. Add the pork to the stockpot. Reduce the heat and leave to simmer for 2 hours.

4. Leave the pork to cool, then cut into cubes.

5. To make the salad, combine extra spring onions with the apple and coriander. Season with salt, lemon juice and oil.

6. Serve the pork belly with the apple salad and a spoonful of stock.

Keto Autumn Vegetable Salad with Saffron Dressing

Difficulty: Easy ¦ Calories: 167 ¦ Serves: 6
Carbs: 9 g ¦ Fat: 12 g ¦ Protein: 3 g

INGREDIENTS

- 12 rainbow carrots, peeled
- 8 stalks long-stem broccoli, halved lengthways
- ½ cucumber cut lengthwise
- 1 medium courgette, sliced
- 4 spring onions, sliced

- 100 g mixed cherry tomatoes, halved
- 3 plum tomatoes, peeled and cut into pieces
- 1 tbsp rapeseed oil
- 30 g black olives, stoned and sliced
- 3 tbsp basil, roughly chopped

DRESSING

- 50 ml extra virgin rapeseed oil
- 20 ml cider vinegar
- 1 tsp caster sugar

- ½ tsp Dijon mustard
- 1 small shallot, chopped
- 1 pinch of saffron strands

PREPARATION

1. Heat a pan over medium heat. Stir in the courgette, carrots and broccoli in rapeseed oil. Stir-fry for 3 minutes, then transfer to a bowl.

2. Add the remaining salad ingredients in a bowl and toss together.

3. To make the dressing, whisk the sugar, saffron, vinegar and mustard together. Season with a pinch of salt and keep whisking until the sugar dissolves. Add in the oil gradually, then the shallots.

4. Serve the salad tossed with the dressing.

Tomato, Burrata and Bean Salad

Difficulty: Easy ¦ Calories: 409 ¦ Serves: 4
Carbs: 7 g ¦ Fat: 32 g ¦ Protein: 22 g

INGREDIENTS

- 500 g tomatoes
- 2 x 100 g burrata
- 150 g broad beans, podded
- 50 g hazelnuts, toasted and chopped
- ½ tsp caster sugar
- 1 tbsp lovage
- 1 tbsp tarragon
- 1 tbsp red wine vinegar
- 2 tsp Dijon mustard
- 3 tbsp olive oil
- 1 tbsp mint leaves
- The zest of 1 lemon
- 1 pinch of fennel seeds
- Handful flat-leaf parsley
- Handful basil

PREPARATION

1. Cut the tomatoes into wedges, and transfer to a bowl. Toss with a pinch of salt and the sugar. Leave to marinate for ½ hour.

2. Meanwhile, bring a pan of water to the boil and cook the beans for 2 minutes. Drain well and allow to cool.

3. Peel the beans out of their shells.

4. Chop the herbs and add into the bowl with the tomatoes. With the mustard, lemon zest, fennel seeds, olive oil and the red wine vinegar. Season with salt if necessary and add in the beans.

5. Transfer to a serving plate. Top with the burrata and the beans. Scatter over the hazelnuts and extra lemon zest if you want.

Asparagus Salad with Poached Egg

Difficulty: Easy ¦ Calories: 228 ¦ Serves: 2
Carbs: 13 g ¦ Fat: 13 g ¦ Protein: 13 g

INGREDIENTS

- 8 asparagus spears, trimmed
- 2 large eggs
- 200 g cooked beetroot, peeled and cut into pieces
- ¼ cucumber, cut into batons
- 1 tbsp balsamic vinegar
- 1 tbsp extra virgin olive oil
- 2 handfuls mixed leaves

PREPARATION

1. Pour the vinegar and olive oil into a small bowl. Add in the beetroot and mix well.
2. Divide the cucumber and mixed leaves into 2 serving plates.
3. Cook the asparagus in simmering water for a couple of minutes.
4. Crack the eggs into a hot pan and cook for a few minutes, until the yolks are just beginning to set.
5. Add the eggs to the salad, pour over the dressing and top with asparagus and a poached egg.

Keto Shrimpo de Gallo

Difficulty: Easy ¦ Calories: 275 ¦ Serves: 8
Carbs: 16 g ¦ Fat: 23 g ¦ Protein: 24 g

INGREDIENTS

- 500 g large shrimps, tails removed
- 1 clove garlic, minced
- 1 avocado, diced
- ½ white onion, chopped
- 30 g chopped cilantro
- 500 g tomatoes, diced
- 1 tbsp extra virgin olive oil
- 2 tbsp fresh lime juice
- ¼ tsp chilli powder
- 2 jalapeno peppers, seeds removed, diced

PREPARATION

1. Heat the oil in a large skillet over medium heat. Cook the shrimps and season with garlic and chilli powder. Transfer to a cutting board.

2. Roughly chop the shrimps into small pieces and transfer into a bowl. Add in the onion, tomatoes, cilantro, lime juice, jalapeno and avocado. Season with salt and pepper to taste.

3. Mix well and serve.

Parmesan and Brussel Sprouts Salad

Difficulty: Easy ¦ Calories: 269 ¦ Serves: 6
Carbs: 12 g ¦ Fat: 19 g ¦ Protein: 16 g

INGREDIENTS

- 900 g Brussel sprouts, halved and sliced
- 130 g freshly chopped parsley
- 5 tbsp lemon juice
- 5 tbsp extra virgin olive oil
- 60 g pomegranate seeds
- 60 g chopped toasted almonds
- Shaved parmesan, to serve

PREPARATION

1. Whisk the oil, lemon juice, parsley, salt and pepper in a bowl.
2. Add in the Brussel sprouts and toss until well coated. Let sit for at least 20 minutes.
3. Add in the pomegranate seeds and almonds.
4. Serve with shaved parmesan.

Keto Strawberry and Spinach Salad

Difficulty: Easy ¦ Calories: 199 ¦ Serves: 4
Carbs: 12 g ¦ Fat: 23 g ¦ Protein: 18 g

INGREDIENTS

- 250 g baby spinach
- ¼ red onion, sliced
- 50 g feta, crumbled
- 10 g chopped toasted pecans
- 2 chicken breasts, cooked and cut into pieces

- 2 tbsp fresh lemon juice
- 1 tbsp extra virgin olive oil
- ½ tsp Dijon mustard
- 120 g strawberries, thinly sliced

PREPARATION

1. Whisk the lemon juice and the mustard in a bowl. Pour in the oil and mix the dressing until well combined.

2. Add in the chicken, spinach, strawberries, ½ of the pecans, and onion. Toss to combine with the dressing.

3. Transfer to serving plates and serve with the remaining pecans and crumbling feta.

Keto Caprese Salad

Difficulty: Easy ¦ Calories: 174 ¦ Serves: 4-6
Carbs: 7 g ¦ Fat: 13 g ¦ Protein: 21 g

INGREDIENTS

- ◆ 450 g fresh mozzarella
- ◆ 6 medium ripe tomatoes, sliced
- ◆ 1 bunch fresh basil, stems removed
- ◆ 1 tbsp extra virgin olive oil

PREPARATION

1. Layer the mozzarella and tomato slices on a large serving plate.

2. Drizzle with olive oil.

3. Season with salt and pepper.

Keto Crispy Pork Belly Salad with Mint and Coriander

Difficulty: Easy ¦ Calories: 389 ¦ Serves: 4
Carbs: 19 g ¦ Fat: 33 g ¦ Protein: 26 g

INGREDIENTS

- 1 kg boneless pork belly, with skin, scored at 1 cm intervals all over
- 1 small cucumber, sliced
- 3 spring onions, sliced
- 1 red chilli, seeds removed, chopped
- 2 tbsp lime juice
- ¼ cup basil leaves
- ¼ cup mint leaves
- 2 tbsp chopped salted peanuts
- ¼ coriander leaves
- 2 tbsp fish sauce
- 2 tsp caster sugar

PREPARATION

1. Preheat the oven to 200 C.
2. Remove excess moisture from the pork skin with a paper towel, then rub all over with salt.
3. Place the pork skin-side up in a roasting pan, cover with water and roast for 2 hours, covering with additional water if necessary. Once ready, set the pork aside and allow to cool, then cut the meat into bite-sized pieces.
4. In a bowl, mix the lime juice, sugar and fish sauce, until the sugar dissolves. Add in the pork, cucumber, spring onion, chilli and herbs. Toss to combine well.
5. Serve the salad with scattered peanuts.

Seared Tuna and Cucumber Salad

Difficulty: Medium ¦ Calories: 254 ¦ Serves: 6-8
Carbs: 9 g ¦ Fat: 11 g ¦ Protein: 29 g

INGREDIENTS

- 400 g ycllowfin tuna steaks
- 2 tbsp sesame oil
- 1 tbsp sunflower oil

- 3 tbsp soy sauce
- 1 tbsp cracked black pepper

SALAD

- 3 cucumber, peeled, halved, and spiralised
- 8 breakfast radishes, trimmed and sliced
- 1 mooli, peeled and spiralised (or use 2 extra breakfast radishes)
- 1 small piece ginger, peeled and cut into matchsticks

- 2 sheets nori, cut into strips
- 3 tbsp mirin
- 1 red chilli, deseeded and chopped
- 1 tbsp coriander seeds, toasted and crushed
- 1 large bunch coriander, chopped
- 2 tbsp sushi ginger, chopped (optional)

DRESSING

- 1 tsp soy sauce
- 4 tbsp natural full-fat yoghurt
- The juice of 1 lime
- 1 tsp wasabi

PREPARATION

1. Whisk the sesame oil, soy sauce and pepper together.

2. Heat the sunflower oil in a frying pan and sear the tuna steaks on both sides until well cooked. Transfer to the sesame oil mixture and leave to marinate for 1 h. Turn the steaks and continue to chill.

3. Meanwhile, to make the salad, mix all the vegetables into a large bowl. Add the ginger and the nori. Drizzle over the lime juice and mirin, then add in the chilli and coriander.

4. To make the dressing, whisk all ingredients together.

5. Serve the tuna with the salad drizzled over with the dressing, and sprinkle over the coriander seeds.

Barbecued Bavette Steak and Tomato Salad

Difficulty: Medium ¦ Calories: 253 ¦ Serves: 6-8
Carbs: 6 g ¦ Fat: 16 g ¦ Protein: 19 g

INGREDIENTS

- 500 g mixed heritage tomatoes
- 200 g grilled artichokes in oil, drained
- 500 g bavette steak

- 150 g feta, crumbled
- 2 tbsp olive oil
- 2 red onions, cut into slices
- ½ bunch chives, shipped

DRESSING

- 3 spring onions, sliced
- 2 tbsp red wine vinegar

- 3 tbsp olive oil
- 1 tsp onion seeds

PREPARATION

1. To make the dressing, whisk the onion seeds, vinegar, spring onions in a bowl.

2. Slice the tomatoes and transfer to a serving platter. Season with salt and drizzle with some oil.

3. Heat a pan and cook the steak for 2-3 minutes on each side. Leave to rest on a plate.

4. Drizzle the remaining oil over the onions, separated into rings, and grill for a few minutes.

5. Slice the steak and serve with the tomatoes over it. Drizzle with the resting juice and top with onions, artichokes, feta and chives. Serve with the dressing.

Keto Chicken Souvlaki with Greek Salad

Difficulty: Challenging ¦ Calories: 279 ¦ Serves: 4
Carbs: 15 g ¦ Fat: 16 g ¦ Protein: 17 g

INGREDIENTS

- 8 boneless chicken thighs, skin on, cut into cubes
- Salt and pepper
- Lemon wedges, to serve

KETO TZATZIKI

- 200 g coconut yoghurt
- ½ cucumber, grated
- 1 tbsp mint leaves, finely chopped
- 1 tbsp extra virgin olive oil
- 1 garlic clove, finely grated
- 1 tsp dill fronds, finely chopped
- 1 tsp lemon juice

MARINADE

- The juice of 2 lemon
- 3 tbsp coconut oil, melted
- 1 tbsp red wine vinegar
- ½ tsp sweet paprika
- 1 tbsp garlic, finely grated
- 1 tsp ground cumin
- 1 tsp dried thyme
- 2 ½ tsp dried oregano
- 1 tsp honey (optional)

GREEK SALAD

- 1 cucumber, halved and sliced
- ¼ red onion, sliced
- 2 tomatoes, cut into wedges
- 1 baby lettuce, quartered
- 3 tbsp extra virgin olive oil
- 2 tbsp red wine vinegar

COCONUT YOGURT

- 1.2 l coconut cream
- 1 tbsp powdered gelatine
- 2 tbsp filtered water
- 4 probiotic capsules
- 1 tbsp lemon juice (optional)
- 2 tbsp honey or coconut sugar (optional)

1. Start with the coconut yoghurt. Wash and prepare a 1.5 l preserving jar with a lid. Place the water in a bowl and sprinkle over the gelatine. Leave to soak for 2 minutes. Heat the vanilla seeds and coconut cream in a saucepan. Stir often until it starts to simmer. Remove from the pan and set aside to cool. Pour 125 ml of this coconut cream into a sterilised bowl and stir in the probiotic powder from the capsules and the lemon juice. Add the remaining mixture and stir well. Pour everything into the jar, seal with the lid and leave to ferment in a warm place for at least 12 hours. Once ready, stir well and refrigerate for at least 5 hours.

2. To make the tzatziki, combine all the ingredients in a bowl and season with salt if needed. Cover and place in the fridge for a few minutes.

3. To make the marinade, combine all the ingredients. Season with salt and pepper.

4. Add the chicken cubes to the marinade and mix until well coated. Place in the fridge and leave to marinate for 2 hours.

5. Once ready, thread the marinated chicken onto some wooden or bamboo skewers. Season with salt and pepper.

6. Cook on a chargrill pan or barbecue grill plate for 15 minutes or until cooked through.

7. Make the salad by mixing all the ingredients in a bowl.

8. Serve the chicken skewers with all the other sauces and the yoghurt, plus extra lemon wedges and the Greek salad.

Keto Indulgent Treats

Keto Cheesecake Fat Bombs

Difficulty: Easy ¦ Calories 50 ¦ Servings 26
Total Carb: 0.5 g ¦ Total Fat: 6 g ¦ Protein: 1 g

INGREDIENTS

- 225 g (8 oz.) cream cheese
- Fresh strawberries
- ¼ cup confectioners swerve
- 6 tbsp salted butter
- Vanilla extract

PREPARATION

1. Microwave the cream cheese for a few seconds, until very soft.
2. Blend or mash the strawberries until pureed. Add vanilla extract and sweetener, and stir well.
3. Combine the strawberry mixture with the butter and the cream cheese. Beat the mixture with a mixer until well-mixed.
4. Scoop the batter into round silicone moulds.
5. Freeze your fat bombs for a couple of hours.
6. Serve frozen.

Low-carb Eggplant Pizza

Difficulty: Medium ¦ Calories 671 ¦ Servings 4
Total Carb: 13 g ¦ Total Fat: 50 g ¦ Protein: 37 g

INGREDIENTS

- 325 g (3/4 lb) ground beef
- 2 eggplants
- Olive oil, for frying
- 175 ml (3/4 cup) tomato sauce
- 275 g (10 oz.) shredded cheese
- 60 g (1/4 cup) chopped fresh oregano
- 1 yellow onion
- ½ tsp ground cinnamon
- Salt and pepper

PREPARATION

1. Preheat the oven to 200 C (400 F)
2. Slice the eggplants, coat with olive oil and bake for 20 minutes.
3. Meanwhile, fry the onion and onion in the remaining olive oil. Add beef and tomato sauce and let simmer for 10 minutes. Season with salt and pepper, if needed.
4. Spread the beef mixture on top of the eggplant slices.
5. Sprinkle with fresh oregano and shredded cheese.
6. Place in the oven until the cheese has melted.

Keto Buffalo Drumsticks with Chili

Difficulty: Medium ¦ Calories 569 ¦ Servings 4
Total Carb: 2 g ¦ Total Fat: 42 g ¦ Protein: 42 g

INGREDIENTS

- 900 g (2 lbs) chicken drumsticks
- 2 tbsp white wine vinegar
- Olive or coconut oil
- 1 tbsp tomato paste
- 1 garlic clove (minced)
- Paprika powder
- Tabasco
- 75 ml (1/3 cup) mayonnaise
- Butter or olive oil, for frying

PREPARATION

1. Preheat oven to 220 C (450 F).
2. Mix all the herbs and spices in a bowl and pour into a plastic bag.
3. Add the chicken drumsticks and shake the bag thoroughly.
4. Let the chicken marinate in the spice's mixtures for 10 minutes.
5. Put the chicken drumsticks in a baking dish and bake for 40 minutes.
6. In a small bowl, mix garlic, chilli and mayonnaise, and serve it with your chicken drumsticks.

Keto Slow-Cooked Pork Roast with Creamy Gravy

Difficulty: Medium ¦ Calories 589 ¦ Servings 6
Total Carb: 3 g ¦ Total Fat: 51 g ¦ Protein: 28 g

INGREDIENTS

PORK ROAST

- 900 g (2 lbs) pork roast
- 600 ml (2 ½ cups) water
- 350 ml (1 ½ cups) gravy
- 5 black peppercorns
- 2 garlic cloves
- 2 tsp dried rosemary or dried thyme
- 40 g (1.5 oz.) fresh ginger
- 1 tbsp paprika powder
- Olive oil or coconut oil
- 1 bay leaf
- Salt and pepper

PREPARATION

1. Preheat oven to 100 C (200 F).
2. Place the meat in a baking dish, add water to cover 1/3 of it.
3. Season with salt and add peppercorns, rosemary (or thyme) and bay leaf.
4. Let it cook for at least 8 hours, covered with aluminium foil.
5. If you are using a slow cooker, you can cook it for 8 hours on low or 4 hours on high. In this case, you will need less water.
6. Once the meat is ready, save the pan juice in a separate pan.
7. Preheat the oven to 220 C (450 F).
8. In a small bowl, add oil, pepper, herbs, garlic and grated ginger.
9. Rub the pork roast with this mixture and then return to the oven for a15 minutes.
10. Serve the pork roast with gravy and a side dish of your choice.

Keto Garlic Knots

Difficulty: Medium ¦ Calories 180 ¦ Servings 8
Total Carb: 4.5 g ¦ Total Fat: 15 g ¦ Protein: 9 g

INGREDIENTS

- 170 g (6 oz.) shredded mozzarella cheese
- 85 g (3 oz.) almond flour
- 1 large egg
- 60 g (2 oz.) cream cheese
- Dried oregano leaves
- Baking powder
- Garlic powder
- Salt and pepper

TOPPINGS

- 1 tbsp butter
- 3 cloves garlic (minced)
- Finely grated parmesan cheese

PREPARATION

1. Preheat the oven to 180 C (360 F).
2. Mix all dry ingredients.
3. Add cream cheese and mozzarella cheese. Microwave until both ingredients are melted.
4. Process the mixture to form a smooth dough.
5. Add the egg, and mix well.
6. Cut the dough and roll each piece to form a knot-like shape.
7. Place all your knots on a greased baking sheet and bake for 15 minutes.
8. While the knots are in the oven, you can prepare the toppings. Mix minced garlic and melted butter.
9. When the knots are ready, brush the garlic butter over each piece and sprinkle parmesan cheese.

Keto Pizza

Difficulty: Challenging ¦ Calories 210 (each slice) ¦ Servings 6
Total Carb: 3.5 g ¦ Total Fat: 17 g ¦ Protein: 13 g

INGREDIENTS

CRUST

- 60 g (2 oz.) cream cheese
- 90 g (3.1 oz.) almond flour
- Shredded mozzarella cheese
- 1 large egg
- Salt and pepper
- Your choice of toppings

PREPARATION

1. Preheat oven to 200 C (400 F).
2. Stir together almond flour, mozzarella cheese and salt.
3. Add cream cheese and microwave until melted.
4. Stir the mixture to form a smooth dough.
5. Place the dough onto a baking sheet or a pizza plate.
6. Cover it with plastic cling wrap and, with your hands, press to spread out to form a thin circle. Pock a few holes with a form over the crust.
7. Bake for 12 minutes.
8. Add toppings of choice and bake until cheese is melted and toppings are cooked.

Keto Mini Cheesecake

Difficulty: Challenging ¦ Calories 230 ¦ Servings 12
Total Carb: 4 g ¦ Total Fat: 23 g ¦ Protein: 5 g

INGREDIENTS

CRUST

♦ 85 g (3 oz.) almond flour

♦ 10 g (0.4 oz.) confectioners swerve sweetener

♦ 3 tbsp salted butter (melted)

FILLING

♦ 225 g (8 oz.) cream cheese

♦ 2 large eggs

♦ 85 g (3 oz.) confectioners swerve sweetener

♦ ¼ cup heavy whipping cream

♦ Vanilla extract

♦ Fresh lemon juice

♦ Fresh raspberries

CRUST

1. Grease 12 silicone baking cups or cupcake tins.
2. Preheat oven to 175 C (350 F).
3. Mix the sweetener and the melted butter. Add the flour and stir to form a dough.
4. Divide the tough amount into your baking cups and bake for 5 minutes.

FILLING

1. Mix the sweetener and the cream cheese with a hand mixer.
2. Had lemon juice, vanilla extract and heavy cream. Process on low speed for 30 seconds.
3. Add eggs, one at a time. Mix well but avoid overmixing the eggs.
4. Add the raspberries and stir with a spatula.
5. Pour the batter among the cupcakes and flatten the surface with a spatula.
6. Bake the mini cheesecakes for 20 minutes.

28 Days Weight Loss Challenge

DAY 1

Breakfast: Keto Butter Cookies (See page 39)

Lunch: Keto Hamburger Patties with Tomato Sauce and Fried Cabbage (See page 61)

Dinner: Low-Carb Bacon Cheeseburger Wraps

Difficulty: Easy ¦ Calories 684¦ Servings 4
Total Carb: 5 g ¦ Total Fat: 51 g ¦ Protein: 48 g

INGREDIENTS

- 200 g (7 oz.) bacon
- 650 g (22 oz.) ground beef
- 10 cherry tomatoes
- 110 g (4 oz.) shredded cheddar cheese

- 110 g (4 oz.) mushrooms
- 1 iceberg lettuce
- Salt and pepper

PREPARATION

1. Cook the bacon.
2. Slice the mushrooms and cook them in the same pan for 5 minutes.
3. Add ground beef and keep cooking. Season with salt and pepper.
4. Wash the iceberg lettuce and separate each leaf.
5. Spoon the beef mixture into lettuce leaves.
6. Sprinkle with cheddar cheese and add sliced cherry tomatoes.

DAY 2

Breakfast: Keto Butter Cookies (See page 39)

Lunch: Keto Salmon Burger with Green Mash

Difficulty: Medium ¦ Calories 1030 ¦ Servings 4
Total Carb: 7 g ¦ Total Fat: 91 g ¦ Protein: 45 g

INGREDIENTS

SALMON BURGERS

- 650 (1 ½ lbs) salmon
- ½ yellow onion
- 1 medium egg
- Salt and pepper

GREEN MASH

- 150 g (5 oz.) butter
- 450 g (1 lb) broccoli florets
- 50 g (2 oz.) grated parmesan cheese

PREPARATION

1. Cut the salmon in small pieces.
2. Preheat the oven to 110 C (220 F).
3. Place the fish and the other burgers ingredients in a food processor and mix until coarse.
4. Shape your burgers and fry them for 5 minutes on each side.
5. To prepare the green mash, you need to chop the broccoli florets into small pieces.
6. Boil the broccoli and, with an immersion blender, mix the florets with butter and parmesan cheese.
7. Season both the salmon and the green mash with salt and pepper and place on a serving plate.

Dinner: Keto Chicken with Lemon and Butter (See page 64)

DAY 3

Breakfast: Keto Almond Flour Biscuits Recipe (See page 41)

Lunch: Keto Hamburger with Creamy Tomato Sauce and Fried Cabbage (See page 61)

Dinner: Keto Prosciutto Wrapped Salmon Skewers

Difficulty: Easy ¦ Calories 680 ¦ Servings 4
Total Carb: 1 g ¦ Total Fat: 62 g ¦ Protein: 28 g

INGREDIENTS

- 450 g (1 lb) salmon
- 100 g (3.5 oz.) prosciutto slices
- 60 g (1/4 cup) finely chopped fresh basil
- Olive oil
- Salt and pepper
- Mayonnaise for serving
- 8 wooden skewers

PREPARATION

1. Cut the salmon pieces lengthwise and mount them on your wooden skewers.
2. Season with salt and pepper, and chopped basil.
3. Wrap one prosciutto slice around each skewer.
4. Cover in olive oil and cook in the oven or on the grill.
5. Serve with mayonnaise or your choice of side dishes.

DAY 4

Breakfast: Keto Western Omelette (See page 38)

Lunch: Keto Baked Salmon with Pesto

Difficulty: Easy | Calories 1025 | Servings 4
Total Carb: 3 g | Total Fat: 88 g | Protein: 52 g

INGREDIENTS

- 900 g (2 lbs) fresh salmon
- 8 tbsp pesto
- 125 ml Greek yoghurt
- 225 ml (1 cup) mayonnaise
- Salt and pepper

PREPARATION

1. Place the salmon in a baking dish.
2. Spread the pesto on top of the salmon.
3. Season with salt and pepper.
4. Bake at 200 C (400 F) for ½ hour.
5. Meanwhile, stir the remaining pesto, to yoghurt and the mayonnaise together.
6. Serve the salmon with the delicious green pesto sauce.

Dinner: Keto Chicken Salad with Avocado and Bacon (See page 56)

DAY 5

Breakfast: Keto Peanut Butter Cookies (See page 40)

Lunch: Keto Pimiento Cheese Meatballs

Difficulty: Easy ¦ Calories 651 ¦ Servings 4
Total Carb: 1 g ¦ Total Fat: 52 g ¦ Protein: 41 g

INGREDIENTS

- 650 g (1 ½ lbs) ground beef
- 75 ml (1/3 cup) mayonnaise
- 1 tsp paprika or chilli powder
- 110 g (4 oz.) cheddar cheese
- 1 egg
- 60 g (1/4 cup) pimientos or pickled jalapeños
- Cayenne pepper
- Mustard
- Butter, for frying
- Salt and pepper

PREPARATION

1. Mix all the ingredients in a bowl.
2. Stir well with a wooden spoon and then, with wet hands, form large meatballs.
3. Fry the meatballs in butter or oil.
4. Serve with mayonnaise, green salad or your choice of side dishes.

Dinner: Keto Chicken Salad with Avocado and Bacon (See page 56)

DAY 6

Breakfast: Keto Coconut Porridge (See page 36)

Lunch: Low-carb Eggplant Pizza (See page 101)

Dinner: Chorizo with Creamed Green Cabbage

Difficulty: Easy ¦ Calories 1276 ¦ Servings 4
Total Carb: 12 g ¦ Total Fat: 115 g ¦ Protein: 46 g

INGREDIENTS

- 650 g (1 ½ lbs) green cabbage
- 650 g (1 ½ lbs) chorizo
- 350 ml (1 ½ cups) heavy whipping cream
- 125 ml (½ cup) fresh parsley
- 60 g (2 oz.) butter
- Lemon zest
- Salt and pepper

PREPARATION

1. Fry the chorizo in butter.
2. Shred the cabbage and add to the pan.
3. Stir the two ingredients for a few minutes, then add heavy whipping cream and let simmer.
4. Add lemon zest and parsley, and season with salt and pepper.

DAY 7

Breakfast: Low Carb Pumpkin Cheesecake Bars (See page 42)

Lunch: Keto Turkey with Cream-Cheese Sauce

Difficulty: Easy ¦ Calories 815 ¦ Servings 4
Total Carb: 7 g ¦ Total Fat: 67 g ¦ Protein: 47 g

INGREDIENTS

- 650 g (1 ½ lbs) turkey breast
- 200 g (7 oz.) cream cheese
- 475 ml (2 cups) heavy whipping cream
- 40 g (1 ½ oz.) small cappers
- Soy sauce
- Butter
- Salt and pepper

PREPARATION

1. Preheat oven to 175 C (350 F).
2. Season the turkey with salt and pepper.
3. Use half of the butter to fry the turkey breast. After a few minutes, move the meat to the oven and finish it off.
4. Pour turkey drippings in a saucepan and add cream cheese and whipping cream.
5. Stir and, with it boils, add soy sauce.
6. Use the remaining butter to sauté the capers.
7. Serve the meat with the cream cheese sauce and fried capers.

Dinner: Keto Turkey Burgers with Tomato Butter (See page 63)

DAY 8

Breakfast: Keto Almond Flour Pancakes (See page 37)

Lunch: Keto Oven Baked Chicken Breasts (See page 54)

Dinner: Low-Carb Vietnamese Pho

Difficulty: Challenging ¦ Calories 459 ¦ Servings 4
Total Carb: 13 g ¦ Total Fat: 25 g ¦ Protein: 40 g

INGREDIENTS

BROTH

♦ 1.8 kg (4 lbs) beef bones and pigs' feet

♦ 4 whole star anise

♦ 2 medium yellow onions

♦ 5 whole cloves

♦ 60 ml (¼ cup) fish sauce

♦ 3 cinnamon sticks

♦ 50 g (2 oz.) fresh ginger

♦ Water

♦ Salt

PHO

♦ 1 lime

♦ 75 g (3 oz.) coconut aminos

♦ 450 g (1 lb) beef

♦ 125 ml (½ cup) bean sprouts

♦ 1 cup green cabbage

♦ 1 scallion

PREPARATION

1. Broil the ginger and onion, then peel the ginger and rinse well.

2. Heat for 2 minutes the star anise, cloves and cinnamon.

3. Add the beef bones and pigs' feet, ginger, onion, fish sauce, water and salt, and bring to a boil.

4. To prepare the ingredients for the pho, slice the cabbage very thinly.

5. Slice the beef and serve on top of the cabbage. Add the sliced scallions and bean sprouts.

6. Add coconut aminos and lime wedges.

DAY 9

Breakfast: Keto Eggs Butter with Smoked Salmon and Avocado

Difficulty: Easy ¦ Calories 1148 ¦ Servings 2
Total Carb: 5 g ¦ Total Fat: 112 g ¦ Protein: 26 g

INGREDIENTS

- 4 eggs
- 2 avocados
- 110 g (4 oz.) smoked salmon
- 150 g (5 oz.) butter
- Olive oil
- Fresh parsley (chopped)
- Salt and pepper

PREPARATION

1. Boil and peel the eggs, then chop them finely.
2. Let the butter rest at room temperature, then mix it with the eggs. Season with salt and pepper, or your choice of spices.
3. Serve the eggs with diced avocado, smoked salmon and parsley. Season with olive oil.

Lunch: Keto Chicken Garam Masala (See page 57)

Dinner: Low Carb Bacon Tenderloin with Roasted Garlic Mash (See page 59)

Breakfast: Keto Mexican Scrambled Eggs

Difficulty: Easy ¦ Calories 229 ¦ Servings 4
Total Carb: 2 g ¦ Total Fat: 18 g ¦ Protein: 14 g

INGREDIENTS

- 6 eggs
- 75 g (3 oz.) shredded cheese
- 30 g (1 oz.) butter
- 1 scallion
- 2 pickled jalapenos
- 1 tomato
- Salt and pepper

PREPARATION

1. Fry the jalapenos, finely chopped tomato and scallion in butter for 3 minutes
2. Whisk the eggs and pour into the pan.
3. Scramble the eggs for a couple of minutes.
4. Add some shredded cheese, salt and pepper.

Lunch: Keto Hamburger Patties with Tomato Sauce and Fried Cabbage (See page 61)

Dinner: Keto Buffalo Drumsticks with Chilli (See page 102)

DAY 11

Breakfast: (See page 38)

Lunch: Keto Asian Meatballs with Thai Basil Sauce

Difficulty: Medium ¦ Calories 858 ¦ Servings 4
Total Carb: 9 g ¦ Total Fat: 79 g ¦ Protein: 29 g

INGREDIENTS

MEATBALLS

- 550 g (1 ¼ lb) ground pork
- 550 g (1 ¼ lbs) green cabbage
- ½ yellow onion
- 1 tbsp fish sauce

- 50 g (2 oz.) butter
- 1 tbsp fresh ginger
- 4 tbsp coconut oil

THAI BASIL SAUCE

- 50 g (2 oz.) radishes
- 1 tbsp fresh Thai basil

- 175 ml (¾ cup) mayonnaise
- Salt and pepper

PREPARATION

1. Mix all the meatball ingredients and, with wet hands, shape into balls.

2. Fry meatballs in oil.

3. In the same pan, add the shredded cabbage. Season with salt and pepper and stir frequently.

4. Serve the meatball with the cabbage on top.

5. To make the Thai basil sauce, chop radishes finely and mix with the mayonnaise and the Thai basil. Serve with your meatballs.

Dinner: Low-Carb Pork Shoulder Chops with Cauliflower Au Gratin (See page 58)

DAY 12

Breakfast: Keto Banana Bread Muffins (See page 35)

Lunch: Keto Fish Casserole with Mushrooms and Mustard

Difficulty: Medium ¦ Calories 858 ¦ Servings 6
Total Carb: 9 g ¦ Total Fat: 74 g ¦ Protein: 39 g

INGREDIENTS

- 450 g (1 lb) mushrooms
- 650 g (1 ½ lb) broccoli or cauliflower florets
- 650 g (1 ½ lb) white fish
- 475 ml (2 cups) heavy whipping cream
- 100 g (3.5 oz.) butter
- 225 g (8 oz.) shredded cheese
- 2 tbsp mustard
- 2 tbsp fresh parsley
- 100 g (3.5 oz.) olive oil
- Salt and pepper

PREPARATION

1. Preheat oven to 175 C (350 F).

2. Cut the mushrooms and fry in butter. Season with salt and pepper, and parsley.

3. Add the mustard and heavy cream and let simmer for 5 minutes.

4. Place the fish in a baking dish. Sprinkle with part of the cheese and pour the mushrooms cream on top. Sprinkle the remaining cheese.

5. Bake for ½ hour.

6. Meanwhile, boil the cauliflower or broccoli florets. Season with olive oil and mash with a spoon or fork.

7. Serve the cauliflower mash with the fish.

Dinner: Keto Pizza (See page 105)

DAY 13

Breakfast: Keto Coconut Porridge (See page 36)

Lunch: Keto Slow-Cooked Pork Roast with Creamy Gravy (See page 103)

Dinner: Keto Pesto Chicken Casserole with Feta and Olives

Difficulty: Easy ¦ Calories 1018 ¦ Servings 4
Total Carb: 6 g ¦ Total Fat: 93 g ¦ Protein: 38 g

INGREDIENTS

- 650 g (1 ½ lbs) boneless chicken thighs
- 400 ml (1 ¼ cups) heavy whipping cream
- 150 g (5 oz.) feta cheese
- 75 g (3 oz.) pitted olives
- 2 tbsp butter
- 5 tbsp red or green pesto
- 1 garlic clove
- 150 g (5 oz.) leafy greens
- Salt and pepper

PREPARATION

1. Preheat oven to 200 C (400 f)
2. Cut the chicken thighs into small pieces and season with salt and pepper.
3. Fry the chicken in butter and place in a baking dish with olives, garlic and feta cheese.
4. Mix heavy cream and pesto, then pour over the meat.
5. Bake for ½ hour.

Breakfast: Keto Almond Flour Biscuits (See page 41)

Lunch: Keto Chicken Casserole

Difficulty: Medium ¦ Calories 739 ¦ Servings 6
Total Carb: 7 g ¦ Total Fat: 62 g ¦ Protein: 37 g

INGREDIENTS

- 450 g (1 lb) cauliflower florets
- 175 ml (3/4 cup) heavy whipping cream
- 900 g (2 lbs) boneless chicken thighs
- 125 ml (1/2 cup) cream cheese
- 110 g (4 oz.) cherry tomatoes
- 1 leek
- 3 tbsp green pesto
- 200 g (7 oz.) shredded cheese
- 40 g (1.5 oz.) butter
- The juice of ½ lemon
- Salt and pepper

PREPARATION

1. Preheat oven to 200 C (400 F)
2. Mix cream cheese with cream, pesto and lemon juice. Season with salt and pepper.
3. Fry the chicken in butter.
4. Place the chicken in a baking dish. Pour the cream mixture over the meat.
5. Top chicken with cauliflower, tomatoes and leek.
6. Sprinkle shredded cheese on top.
7. Bake for ½ hour.

Dinner: Keto Chicken with Lemon and Butter (See page 64)

DAY 15

Breakfast: Keto Almond Flour Pancakes (See page 37)

Lunch: Keto Thai Fish Curry

Difficulty: Easy | Calories 914 | Servings 4
Total Carb: 10 g | Total Fat: 79 g | Protein: 42 g

INGREDIENTS

- 650 g (1 ½ lbs) salmon
- 475 ml (2 cups) unsweetened coconut cream
- 450 g (1 lb) cauliflower or broccoli florets

- 125 ml (1/2 cup) fresh cilantro
- 4 tbsp red curry paste
- 4 tbsp butter
- 1 tbsp olive oil
- Salt and pepper

PREPARATION

1. Preheat oven to 200 C (400 F).
2. Place the fish in a baking dish greased with olive oil. Season with salt and pepper and add a bit of butter on top of each piece of salmon.
3. Mix the chopped cilantro, coconut cream and curry paste, and pour over the fish.
4. Bake for 20 minutes.
5. Meanwhile, boil the cauliflower or broccoli florets. Serve the vegetables with the fish.

Dinner: Low-carb Eggplant Pizza (See page 101)

Breakfast: Keto Smoked Salmon and Avocado Plate

Difficulty: Easy ¦ Calories 811 ¦ Servings 4
Total Carb: 4 g ¦ Total Fat: 75 g ¦ Protein: 23 g

INGREDIENTS

- ◆ 200 g (7 oz.) smoked salmon
- ◆ 125 ml (1/2 cup) mayonnaise
- ◆ 2 avocados
- ◆ Salt and pepper

PREPARATION

1. Split the avocados in half and scoop out the avocado pieces.

2. Serve the avocados with salmon and a spoonful of mayonnaise.

3. Season with salt and pepper.

Lunch: Keto Super-Easy Stir Fry (See page 55)

Dinner: Keto Turkey Burgers with Tomato Butter (See page 63)

DAY 17

Breakfast: Keto Banana Bread Muffins (See page 35)

Lunch: Keto Grilled Tuna Salad with Garlic Dressing

Difficulty: Easy ¦ Calories 975 ¦ Servings 2
Total Carb: 9 g ¦ Total Fat: 79 g ¦ Protein: 53 g

INGREDIENTS

- 325 g (3/4 lb) tuna (sliced)
- 225 g (8 oz.) green asparagus
- 2 eggs
- 50 g (2 oz.) cherry tomatoes
- 110 g (1/4 lb) leafy greens
- 2 tbsp pumpkin seeds (optional)
- ½ red onion
- 150 ml (2/3 cup) mayonnaise
- Garlic powder
- Salt and pepper

PREPARATION

1. Prepare the garlic dressing by mixing mayonnaise, water, garlic powder and salt and pepper.

2. Boil and peel the eggs.

3. Cut the asparagus into lengths and fry with no oil or butter.

4. Fry or grill the tuna.

5. To make the salad, mix the asparagus, leafy greens, tomatoes and onions. Cut the eggs in half and add to your salad.

6. Slice the tuna and add it to the salad.

7. Pour the dressing and sprinkle with pumpkin seeds (optional).

Dinner: Keto Oven Baked Chicken Breasts (See page 54)

DAY 18

Breakfast: Keto Western Omelette (See page 38)

Lunch: Keto Super-Easy Stir Fry (See page 55)

Dinner: Keto Chicken Cheesesteak Casserole

Difficulty: Medium ¦ Calories 740 ¦ Servings 8
Total Carb: 7 g ¦ Total Fat: 61 g ¦ Protein: 39 g

INGREDIENTS

- 900 g (2 lbs) boneless chicken thighs
- 225 g (8 oz.) mushrooms
- 225 g (8 oz.) cream cheese
- 225 g (8 oz.) cheddar cheese
- 350 g (12 oz.) provolone cheese
- 125 ml (1/2 cup) mayonnaise
- 110 g (4 oz.) yellow onions
- 175 g (6 oz.) green bell peppers
- 2 garlic cloves
- 1 tbsp butter
- 2 tbsp Worcestershire sauce
- 2 tsp Italian seasoning
- Salt and pepper

PREPARATION

1. Preheat oven to 190 C (375 F).

2. Fry the chicken in butter. When the meat is ready, add sliced mushrooms, pepper, onions, and half of the garlic. Season with salt and pepper, and half of the Italian seasoning.

3. In a bowl, mix mayonnaise, cream cheese, the rest of the garlic and the Italian seasoning, cheddar cheese and Worcestershire sauce.

4. Combine this mixture with the meat and place in a baking dish.

5. Top with slices of provolone cheese.

6. Bake for ½ hour.

DAY 19

Breakfast: Keto Coconut Porridge (See page 36)
Lunch: Roasted Pork Belly with Creamed Cabbage

Difficulty: Easy ¦ Calories 1263 ¦ Servings 6
Total Carb: 8 g ¦ Total Fat: 126 g ¦ Protein: 21 g

INGREDIENTS

- ◆ 1.1 kg (2 ½ lbs) pork belly
- ◆ 1 yellow onion
- ◆ ½ tsp cloves
- ◆ 1 tbsp fennel seeds
- ◆ Olive oil
- ◆ Salt and pepper

CREAMED CABBAGE

- ◆ 900 g (2 lbs) cabbage
- ◆ 225 ml (1 cup) heavy whipping cream
- ◆ 50 g (2 oz.) butter
- ◆ 2 tbsp cream cheese
- ◆ Salt and pepper

1. Preheat oven to 175 C (350 F).

2. Make sure that the pork's skin is very dry. With a sharp knife, score it, avoiding to cut the meat.

3. Mix the spices with salt and pepper. Rub the mixture all over the pork belly.

4. Drizzle olive oil and bake the pork for about two hours, depending on its size.

5. Meanwhile, slice the onion and add it to the baking dish.

6. Increase the temperature to 200 C (400 F) and cook for another 30 minutes.

7. While the pork belly is in the oven, you can prepare the cabbage by slicing it and removing the core.

8. Fry the cabbage in butter, and season with salt and pepper.

9. Add cream cheese and cream and let it simmer.

10. Serve the pork belly with the creamed cabbage and slices of baked onion.

Dinner: Keto Hamburger Patties with Tomato Sauce and Fried Cabbage (See page 61)

DAY 20

Breakfast: Keto Butter Cookies (See page 39)

Lunch: Keto Chicken with Lemon and Butter (See page 64)

Dinner: Keto Coconut Salmon with Napa Cabbage

Difficulty: Easy ¦ Calories 764 ¦ Servings 4
Total Carb: 3 g ¦ Total Fat: 68 g ¦ Protein: 32 g

INGREDIENTS

- 550 g (1 ¼ lb) fresh salmon
- 550 g (1 ¼ lb) Napa cabbage
- 50 g (2 oz.) finely shredded coconut (unsweetened)
- 110 g (4 oz.) butter
- Turmeric
- Onion powder
- Salt and pepper
- Olive or coconut oil
- Lemon juice

PREPARATION

1. Cut the salmon in pieces and season with olive or coconut oil.
2. Cut the cabbage in wedges and fry it.
3. Melt the butter and pour it over the salmon and cabbage.
4. Season with salt and pepper, and fresh lemon juice.

Breakfast: Keto Mushroom Omelette

Difficulty: Easy ¦ Calories 517 ¦ Servings 1
Total Carb: 5 g ¦ Total Fat: 44 g ¦ Protein: 26 g

INGREDIENTS

- 3 eggs
- 30 g (1 oz.) shredded cheese
- 4-5 large mushrooms
- ¼ yellow onion
- Butter, for frying
- Salt and pepper

PREPARATION

1. Whisk the egg with salt and pepper until smooth.

2. Chop the onion and fry in butter. Slice the mushrooms and add to the pan, then pour the egg mixture.

3. Sprinkle some cheddar cheese over the egg when they are still hot and a bit raw on top.

4. With a spatula, fold the omelette over in half.

5. Remove from the heat and serve with your choice of sauce.

Lunch: Low Carb Bacon Tenderloin with Roasted Garlic Mash (See page 59)

Dinner: Keto Cornbread (with your choice of side dish) (See page 33)

DAY 22

Breakfast: Keto Scrambled Eggs with Halloumi Cheese

Difficulty: Easy ¦ Calories 517 ¦ Servings 2
Total Carb: 4 g ¦ Total Fat: 59 g ¦ Protein: 28 g

INGREDIENTS

- 75 g (3 oz.) halloumi cheese
- 110 g (4 oz.) bacon
- 50 g (2 oz.) pitted olives
- 4 eggs
- 2 scallions
- Fresh parsley
- Olive oil
- Salt and pepper

PREPARATION

1. Fry the diced halloumi in olive oil with the diced bacon and chopped scallion.

2. Meanwhile, whisk the eggs together and season with parsley, and salt and pepper.

3. Pour the egg mixture over the bacon and cheese.

4. Add the olives and stir well for 2-3 minutes.

Lunch: Keto Frittata with Spinach (See page 29)

Dinner: Keto Chicken Garam Masala (See page 57)

Breakfast: Low Carb Pumpkin Cheesecake Bars (See page 42)

Lunch: Keto Fried Salmon with Green Beans

Difficulty: Easy ¦ Calories 705 ¦ Servings 2
Total Carb: 6 g ¦ Total Fat: 58 g ¦ Protein: 38 g

INGREDIENTS

- ◆ 350 g (12 oz.) fresh salmon
- ◆ 250 g (9 oz.) fresh green beans
- ◆ 75 g (3 oz.) butter
- ◆ ½ lemon juice
- ◆ Salt and pepper

PREPARATION

1. Fry the salmon and the green beans together.
2. Season with salt and pepper and squeeze some fresh lemon juice.

Dinner: Keto Pizza (See page 105)

DAY 24

Breakfast: Keto Western Omelette (See page 38)

Lunch: Japanese Kingfish Lettuce Cups

Difficulty: Easy ¦ Calories 370 ¦ Servings 4
Total Carb: 13 g ¦ Total Fat: 3 g ¦ Protein: 25 g

INGREDIENTS

- 800 g (28.2 oz.) kingfish fillet
- 6 spring onions
- 1 garlic clove
- 2 gem lettuces
- 4 watermelon radishes
- 1 tbsp fish sauce
- 2 tbsp soy sauce
- 2 tbsp peanut or sunflower oil
- Barbecue sauce, for serving

PREPARATION

1. Process the kingfish with a food processor until finely chopped.
2. Fry the onions and garlic in peanut oil. Add the fish and cook for another 2 minutes.
3. Add the fish sauce and soy sauce and stir for 2-3 minutes.
4. Serve the fish mixture in lettuce leaves.
5. Top with radish slices, cabbage and barbecue sauce.

Dinner: Low-Carb Pork Shoulder Chops with Cauliflower Au Gratin (See page 58)

DAY 25

Breakfast: No-Bread Keto Sandwich

Difficulty: Easy ¦ Calories 354 ¦ Servings 2
Total Carb: 2 g ¦ Total Fat: 30 g ¦ Protein: 20 g

INGREDIENTS

- 4 eggs
- 50 g (2 oz.) cheddar cheese
- 2 tbsp butter
- 30 g (1 oz.) smoked ham
- Tabasco or Worcestershire sauce (optional)
- Salt and pepper

PREPARATION

1. Fry the eggs and season with salt and pepper.
2. Place a slice of ham on each egg, using it as the base of a sandwich.
3. Add the cheese and top with another fried egg.
4. Leave the cheese melt on low heat and season with tabasco or Worcestershire sauce.

Lunch: Keto Chicken Salad with Avocado and Bacon (See page 56)

Dinner: Keto Chicken with Lemon and Butter (See page 64)

DAY 26

Breakfast: Keto Western Omelette (See page 38)

Lunch: Keto Frittata with Spinach (See page 29)

Dinner: Goat Cheese and Vegetables Frittata

Difficulty: Easy ¦ Calories 425 ¦ Servings 4
Total Carb: 6 g ¦ Total Fat: 11 g ¦ Protein: 29 g

INGREDIENTS

- 16 eggs
- 300 g (10.5 oz.) soft goat cheese
- 2 bunches broccoli florets
- 2 zucchinis
- 120 g (4.2 oz.) baby peas
- 200 g (7 oz.) mixed cherry tomatoes
- 1 tbsp white wine vinegar
- Finely chopped chives
- Olive oil
- Salt and pepper

PREPARATION

1. Preheat oven to 200 C (400 F).

2. Whisk together the eggs and some water.

3. In a pan, stir in the peas, chives, broccoli florets, half the zucchini (cut into pieces) and ¾ of the goat cheese.

4. Pour the egg mixture and cook for 2-3 minutes.

5. Transfer the frittata to the oven and bake for ½ hour.

6. Meanwhile, make a tomato salad by mixing the halved cherry tomatoes, olive oil and extra chives.

7. Spread the remaining goat cheese over the frittata and serve with tomato salad.

DAY 27

Breakfast: Keto Almond Flour Biscuits (See page 41)

Lunch: Keto Super-Easy Stir Fry (See page 55)

Dinner: Low-Carb Prawns with Buttermilk Dressing and Celery Salad

Difficulty: Easy ¦ Calories 615 ¦ Servings 4
Total Carb: 4 g ¦ Total Fat: 30 g ¦ Protein: 25 g

INGREDIENTS

- 24 large prawns (peeled)
- 2 sticks celery
- Mint leaves
- 1 fennel
- 60 ml (1/4 cup) extra virgin olive oil
- 60 ml (1/4 cup) buttermilk
- 3 garlic cloves
- 1 tsp mustard
- 1 tbsp white wine vinegar
- The juice of 1 lemon
- 1 tbsp finely chopped chives

PREPARATION

1. Brush the prawns with a mixture made of the olive oil, garlic, and lemon juice. Let it marinate for 10-15 minutes.

2. Mix mustard, vinegar, buttermilk, olive oil, chives and season.

3. Combine this mixture with celery leaves, fennel and mint leaves.

4. Cook prawns on a grill or barbecue for 5 minutes and serve with buttermilk dressing and celery salad.

DAY 28

Breakfast: Keto Almond Flour Biscuits Recipe (See page 41)

Lunch: Crisp Pork Belly Salad with Mint and Coriander

Difficulty: Medium ¦ Calories 460 ¦ Servings 4
Total Carb: 4 g ¦ Total Fat: 25 g ¦ Protein: 64 g

INGREDIENTS

- 1 kg (2.2 lbs) boneless pork belly
- 3 spring onions
- 1 long red chilli
- 1 small cucumber
- Fresh mint leaves
- Fresh basil leaves
- Fresh coriander leaves
- 2 tbsp lime juice
- 2 tsp caster sugar
- 2 tbsp fish sauce
- Chopped salted peanuts

PREPARATION

1. Preheat the oven to 200 C (400 F).
2. Rub the pork with salt and place it skin-side up on a roasting pan. Pour in boiling water and roast for 2 hours.
3. When the pork is ready, cut it into bite-sized pieces.
4. Whisk the sugar, fish sauce and lime juice in a bowl.
5. Add the pork, the sliced onion, cucumber, chilli and herbs.
6. Scatter the pork and dressing with peanuts and serve.

Dinner: Keto Pizza (See page 105)

Disclaimer

This book contains opinions and ideas of the author and is meant to teach the reader informative and helpful knowledge while due care should be taken by the user in the application of the information provided. The instructions and strategies are possibly not right for every reader and there is no guarantee that they work for everyone. Using this book and implementing the information/recipes therein contained is explicitly your own responsibility and risk. This work with all its contents, does not guarantee correctness, completion, quality or correctness of the provided information. Misinformation or misprints cannot be completely eliminated.

EXCLUSIVE BONUS

40 Weight Loss Recipes

&

14 Days Meal Plan

Scan the QR-Code and receive
the FREE download:

Printed in Great Britain
by Amazon

16711301R00080